OPEN
& DISTANCE
LEARNING
FOR NURSES

Editied by
Kate Robinson

Longman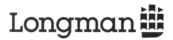

Industry and Public Service Management Division
Longman Group UK Limited
Westgate House, The High, Harlow, Essex CM20 1YR

First Published 1989

British Library Cataloguing in Publication Data

Robinson, Kate
    Open and distance learning for nurses.
    1. Nurses. Professional education. Applications of distance study
    I. Title
    610.73'07'11

ISBN 0-582-04616-5

Typeset by P's & Q's Ltd., 18 Harrington Street, Liverpool L2 9QA
Printed in Great Britain by Bell and Bain Ltd., Glasgow

Contents

Foreword by Dorothy Spencer   v

Authors   vii

Introduction   ix

Acknowledgments   xii

Part 1: Politics and policies

1   Open learning: the current scene   3
Kate Robinson

2   Open learning: definitions and debates   19
Kate Robinson

Part 2: The agony of production

3   Producing materials: an overview   39
Kate Robinson

4   Setting up a production unit: issues and challenges   53
Elisabeth Clark and Kate Robinson

5   TASC analysis: designing and testing an   67
open learning package
John Paley

6   Writing for competencies   86
Barbara Vaughan

7   The role of the open learning editor   103
Jan Fordham

8   Choosing and using media   121
Fiona Munro

Part 3: The ecstacy of delivery

9   Delivering open learning : an overview   139
Kate Robinson

10   Supporting learners in the workplace   152
Steve Wright

11   The Diploma in Nursing: a study centre network   163
Kate Robinson

12 Hybrid courses in continuing professional development   174
    Elisabeth Clark

13 Helping enrolled nurses   189
    Margaret Johnston

14 Helping bank nurses   200
    Wendy Green

15 Highland Health Board: a coordinated scheme   210
    Chris Wakeling

Part 4: Postscript

16 Postscript   227
    Kate Robinson

Further reading   238

Foreword

The development of open and distance learning has been an event of major importance to nursing education. The combination of highly-flexible open learning techniques with specific, professional subject areas for nurses has added a new dimension to the diversifying characterisation of nursing education.

In spite of a landslide of packages and reviews, no books devoted to open and distance learning for nurses have been published until now. The authors have, therefore, found it expedient to try to collect the sum of our present knowledge about application and techniques of open learning in this book.

Initially, Kate Robinson focuses on why open and distance learning has become important and on the developmental role of a number of agencies, emphasising, too, the educational benefits of moving some control to the student in the context of promoting the 'independent practitioner'.

The production of materials, the practical issues of combining the use of learning materials with teaching methodologies and support for the students are comprehensively covered.

Open and distance learning is now becoming a part of established practice in the provision of continuing education to help nurses orientate themselves to specific professional roles; the advantages include consistency of message, large-scale delivery, ease of access, flexible entry and length of programme. The role of the tutor is adapting to focus on the facilitation of open learning alongside other established educational methods.

Open and distance learning has been used in such a diversity of connections that no 'authorised' version of the method exists. The inclusion of a number of authors, all describing a specific area of expertise, especially increases the value of this book. This approach should give tutors seeking facts in this particular sphere a chance to find useful information.

It is hoped that the combination of techniques and applications in one handbook, will, besides illustrating the applicability of open and distance learning, be a source of inspiration to tutors working in other fields.

Dorothy Spencer, BA, RGN, RMN,   July 1989
RCNT, RNT, MBIM
Adviser in Nursing Education Royal College of Nurses
and Chairman of Continuing Nursing Education Advisory
Board for Barnet and Manchester Colleges Open Learning
Initiatives since 1982.

Authors

Fiona Munro
Freelance Consultant; formerly media officer to the Distance Learning Centre at South Bank Polytechnic.

Elisabeth Clark
Director of the Distance Learning Centre, South Bank Polytechnic.

Jan Fordham
Managing Editor, Distance Learning Centre, South Bank Polytechnic; formerly editor of the Open University pack *A Systematic Approach to Nursing Care.*

Wendy Green
Tutor, Clinical Practice Development Team, Oxfordshire Health Authority. Consultant author for the Distance Learning Centre, South Bank Polytechnic.

Margaret Johnston
Nurse Teacher for Enrolled Nurses, Oxfordshire Health Authority

John Paley
Director, Centre for Crime Prevention Studies, Cranfield Institute of Technology, and Director of Social Care Open Learning Ltd.

Kate Robinson
Lecturer in Nursing and Health Studies, Department of Health and Social Welfare, the Open University. Formerly Director of the Distance Learning Centre, South Bank Polytechnic.

Barbara Vaughan
Senior Lecturer in Nursing, Department of Nursing, University of Wales, Cardiff. Consultant author and editor of open learning texts for the Open University, the Distance Learning Centre and the Continuing Nurse Education programme.

Chris Wakeling
Director of Nurse Education, Highland College of Nursing and Midwifery

Steve Wright
Consultant Nurse, Department of Medicine for the Elderly and Nursing Development Unit, Tameside General Hospital. Consultant author for the Continuing Nurse Education Programme.

Introduction

I have envisaged that many of the readers of this book will be teachers of nurses and possibly also of nursing, who are curious about open and distance learning, not yet convinced of its efficacy, but keen to learn more and perhaps experiment more before they make a judgement. Other readers will be managers faced with the challenge of organising education for their nursing staff and keen to learn about any approach which can offer to deliver a complex educational programme, responsive to practice needs and sensitive to the necessity to avoid disrupting patient care.

Although this book is about open and distance learning in nursing, I would be foolish to claim that it covered the whole subject from top to bottom. Open learning - and for reasons which are explained in Chapter 2 this is the preferred term - is far too complex a subject to be dealt with in one book. So this book is not a recipe book in a simplistic sense, but it will help the reader to 'know what it is they need to know', whatever role they envisage taking within an open learning system.

The book is intended to emphasise three themes. First, and most importantly, I have tried to ground the discussion about open learning in time and space. That is to say, I have asked the contributors to talk about their own experiences and their own schemes, which are - as practice always is - grounded in particular needs, problems and potentials. These schemes are not intended to be typical, they are not chosen as a representative sample, but they do offer a vehicle for a discussion of how open learning can offer practical solutions to everyday problems. As such, they cannot be directly translated into your situation, which is unique to you, but they will help you identify the sorts of things which you should be thinking about when introducing open learning. This essentially practical discussion is appropriately based in theory, but hopefully the links between theory and practice are well established. Because the contributors were describing their own individual schemes, the degree to which their work has been placed within the context of open learning theory will vary depending on the nature and purpose of the scheme, but Parts Two and Three begin with an overview which should help place the discussions in context.

Second, there has been an emphasis on the challenges of introducing open learning. The basic thesis is that bringing any aspect of open learning into your existing practice will be a complex and complicated business which will require proper planning and resourcing. Writing open learning materials is a long, often exciting but also tedious exercise, which, if it is to be done properly, requires extensive staff training and adequate resourcing. Similarly, the enrolment of your learners into an open learning system, however informal, will need both a staff training programme and a student training programme. Open learning involves a different way of looking at things, and our eyes need to become accustomed - it is not just a matter of putting on new spectacles. I am reminded of the time when, as a young, and obviously naive, new teacher in further education I tried out my ideas on student autonomy and self-motivation on 'Bricklayers 3'. 'Bricklayers 3' had been used to signing in and out and asking permission before wiping their noses. When I grandly told them that they didn't have to ask permission before leaving class and going to the lavatory they took me at my word. And in the hour I spent outside the men's lavatories begging them to come out, I learnt a great deal about the folly of precipitate change, however worthy the ideology which you are introducing. So our second theme is that open learning is an innovation, and like any innovation it will have intended and unintended consequences, and therefore deserves to be thought through very carefully. It is not an easy option.

The third theme is perhaps a more positive one, and that is that open learning is here to stay. And that assertion rests on the definition of open learning as a philosophy supported by technology rather than just a technology of delivering learning. Chapter 2 explores the concept of open learning rather more closely, but Chapter 1 is also important because it shows that much of the impetus for open learning is coming from outside nursing. Yet Project 2000 demonstrates very well that nursing cannot ignore general developments in vocational education. The decades to come will see nursing tied ever more closely to general educational institutions and ideologies.

The book is organised into four parts based around the division between producing open learning and running an open scheme which is found in the literature. Although many teachers and managers might assume that Part Three on delivering open learning deals most forthrightly with their concerns, a reading of all four parts will give a much broader and deeper understanding of the potential of open learning.

The *first part* is an overview of the history and current ideas and institutions in open and distance learning in the UK. There is particular reference to nursing but it is set in the context of education and training in general.

The *second part* explores the issues of the production of learning materials. I am conscious that most people involved in open learning will be *using* rather than *making* materials, and indeed one of the underlying messages is that the difficulties dictate that production should remain a specialised activity carried on in specialist centres. However, it is important that users understand the complexities of the materials both so that they can distinguish good from bad and so that they can feel more confident in adapting materials to their particular purposes without prejudicing the integrity of the materials.

The *third part* is concerned with the distribution of the materials and the systems needed to support the learners. This important part of open learning is threatened on two sides. First, there are those who want to introduce open learning to save money and therefore want to cut support systems. Second, there are those who are so concerned about learner support that they want to increase it until it matches that offered in conventional education; such people are perhaps more well meaning but have failed to grasp that encouraging learner autonomy must include an element of risk taking.

The *postscript* looks at some of the important issues which a debate on open learning should address, and also proposes that open learning has a potential for emancipation which nursing badly needs to exploit.

Each chapter is free standing so that you can dip into the material as you wish, although there are cross references where they seemed helpful. The book ends with suggestions for further reading, although each chapter is individually referenced.

So, we hope that you will find the book both stimulating and useful. We are conscious that we have only been able to sketch out in broad terms the schemes which we are involved in, but individual approaches for more information will always be welcome. The details of the authors and their institutions are on page vii. We have tried to be enthusiastic but not naive, and have therefore talked about the problems as well as the benefits. Indeed you may well feel that there is such a lot of talk about the difficulties that you are deterred from getting started; this would be a pity as open learning has enormous potential within nurse education.

Kate Robinson
Milton Keynes

Acknowledgments

I would like to thank all those who have agreed to contribute to this book and the many other of my colleagues who have generated my interest in open and distance learning as a topic for debate as well as a task to be done. I would particularly like to acknowledge the contribution of Nick Fox from the Training Commission, Liz Clark from the Distance Learning Centre and Glennis Johnson from the Continuing Nurse Education programme. However the major, unacknowledged, intellectual and practical contribution to the book came from Hugh Robinson, to whom I am very grateful.

Kate Robinson   August 1989

Part 1:
Politics and policies

1 Open learning: the current scene

Kate Robinson

The metaphor of the span of the earth's history as a twenty four hour clock is always impressive – particularly when we discover that human beings have only arrived at the party just before midnight. Suppose that we apply the same metaphor to education – when did open learning come onto the scene? Unlike humanity, open learning arrived earlier than we think. *Pitman's Journal* of 1924 was discussing the value of open and distance learning in terms which would be familiar to many open learning tutors today.

> One of the most recent developments in recent years in the educational world has been the growth of tuition by distance learning... The greatest value is felt by those students who are unable to attend classes or lectures... Tutorial comment and criticism are valuable factors of open learning and... a bond of sympathy between tutor and pupil exists throughout the course.
>
> *Pitman's Journal,* 6 December 1924 (cited in OU1988)

This quotation contains both the relevant terms: *open learning* and *distance learning*. Whether there is any difference between them is a topic which will be explored in the next chapter but, for the sake of brevity rather than as an intellectual statement, the term *open learning* is used throughout the book, unless an author wants to make a particular point about the two terms.

Suppose that we exploit another familiar metaphor and think of the career of open learning in terms of a human lifespan. Is it a wailing insecure infant, a pushy adolescent or a mature adult weighed down with worries about the mortgage? The answer, as with many human beings, is probably a little bit of each, but open learning is certainly well past the stage of infant vulnerability. Ten years ago it might have been possible to imagine the premature death of the infant open learning from a number of causes – lack of parental interest, lack of resources, antagonism from its older and bigger siblings – yet today it is strong and well established, supported at all levels by government encouragement and finance. After a shaky start, open learning has become respectable and acknowledged. Its progress can be documented in a number of ways: the number of institutions wholly concerned with open learning, the number of books published, the number of students enrolled. This latter category affords some very impressive statistics: in the late 1980s the Open University had about 70,000 undergraduate enrolments, and a further 100,000 learners in the continuing education programme, whilst in the mid-1980s the National Extension College had over 10,000 enrolments.

Yet is this picture of encouragement true of open learning in nursing? Has the antagonism towards open learning which was so manifest in the early 1980s given way to enthusiasm, tolerance or does it remain as barely suppressed hatred? Again, there are a number of indicators we could use to support an encouraging answer: the Department of Health funded research study into open learning in nursing, the frequency of references to open learning by the United Kingdom Central Council and the National Boards, the number of articles and supplements appearing in the nursing press, the fact of an open learning version of the Diploma in Nursing successfully launched, and so on. Certainly these all lend credence to the notion that open learning is in nursing to stay.

But how did this heady state of affairs come about from the shaky beginnings of the early 1980s and is it quite as positive as it seems? To understand the present position of open learning in nursing and to speculate on its future, we need to look at how it has come to the position it currently holds and, in particular, at the forces which have guided its progress, both within and without nursing.

There are two sets of factors which are currently moulding the position of open and distance learning in nurse education. The first set are those factors which are extrinsic to nursing, such as the development of open learning initiatives elsewhere in the education system. The second set are those factors which are intrinsic to nursing, such as the development of continuing education for practitioners and the financial framework of nurse education.

Developments outside nursing

The most important institution in the development of open learning in the United Kingdom (and possibly the world) is the Open University. However, it needs be appreciated that the Open University was itself established within the receptive environment created by its predecessor, the National Extension College, which was set up in 1963. In recent years, other initiatives, such as Open Tech and Open College, have joined the scene and begun to influence the way in which we think about open and distance learning.

The National Extension College

A history of the National Extension College (Jenkins and Perraton 1980) is entitled *The Invisible College* and it remains a *relatively* unknown and unacknowledged player in the open learning game, although this invisibility has been ameliorated by the subsequent rising consciousness about open learning and by the publicity attendant on the 25th anniversary of the College (Paine 1988). Nevertheless, it is a major open learning institution in the United Kingdom and its history illustrates a number of the themes of open learning which have been important to subsequent developments.

The founder chairman of the National Extension College (NEC) was Michael Young, who was also the founder of the Consumer Association. This Association had drawn attention to the inadequacies of the existing correspondence colleges, and the NEC can be seen as part of the wider consumer movement of the 1960s. However, although the NEC was intended to remedy the deficiencies of the existing provision, it was not intended to challenge conventional education. It defined its potential students in very limited terms.

> Who are the students – or 'members', as we shall call them – of the College? They will be people who need a second chance – those who did not have the education they would like when they were younger and who are not getting it now, people who want to change their jobs or improve their qualifications in their present careers. Obviously we will not appeal to all such people, and will not even try. Anyone who can get into a university, or even attend classes at a technical college, evening institute or WEA should do so. We are thinking rather of the people who cannot turn up regularly for ordinary classes, above all of married women housebound by their children, or whose job keeps them travelling, those who are on shift-work or tied to a hospital, people who have to study in odd moments of the week if they are to study at all...
>
> Michael Young in 1963 (cited in Jenkins and Perraton 1980)

The idea of a 'second chance' for those who simply could not take advantage of existing provision was clearly an important part of the rationale for the establishment of the NEC, as was the potential of the new technologies of radio and television. The NEC has never had automatic access to these media but the possibility of using them alongside text based materials has been explored at every opportunity (Jenkins and Perraton 1980).

Another of the justifications for the establishment of the NEC was as an experiment which would lay the foundations for a 'University of the Air' (as the Open University was originally conceived) – an idea which was being promoted but was not yet established. In this, as in other aspects of its work, it was successful, although the link between the two institutions is not now as obvious as might be expected.

One of the programmes of the NEC – Flexistudy – involves the NEC producing materials and liaising with a number of colleges to offer face to face tuition in support of the materials. Thus the NEC combined with local colleges to offer the complete service which the NEC felt it could not, or should not, offer alone. Although the courses offered were mainly academic courses such as GCSE and A level, rather than vocational, a number of people in work (including nurses) took them in order to increase their basic academic qualifications; perhaps so that they could subsequently gain entry to a vocational training course.

So, in the history of the NEC we can see most of the basic themes of open learning: the idea of a 'second chance' for those who cannot manage the logistics of conventional courses, the emphasis on matching the standards of conventional courses, the exploitation of the media for education wherever possible, and the collaboration between institutions to offer a complete service to the learner. However, there is no notion that open learning might supplant conventional education or prove superior to it – a notion that was also absent from the early years of the Open University.

The Open University

The Open University has been described as 'Probably the most important and far-reaching experiment in adult education in the last twenty years in Britain...' (Ellwood 1976). The nature of the experiment and the importance of the Open University lies in the the combination of the method of delivery of the teaching, which is wholly by distance teaching methods, within the context of a conventional university institution. The Open University is just that – a university – in every sense of the term, with a full size academic staff involved in teaching and research, and conducting themselves within the confines of a Charter which is surprisingly conventional and similar to that of any other United Kingdom university (Perry 1976).

However, the central part of the Open University programme was (and still is) concerned with a general undergraduate programme which does not offer specialist degrees. There was a small continuing education programme, part of which was concerned with vocational education for health and social care, but the importance of this work was only fully acknowledged in the late 1980s. Such an acknowledgement can be seen as a response to other initiatives in vocational education, such as that of the Open Tech initiative.

The Open Tech initiative

The Open Tech initiative of the Manpower Services Commission (MSC) was designed to promote the use of open learning for the training of the British workforce. As David Tinsley comments,

> MSC's commitment to open learning did not stem from any theoretical commitment to educational philosophy – though many of us who have been involved are excited by the possibilities it opens up. Instead the Commission is concerned with satisfying its practical remit to ensure that British training systems meet the present and future needs of the economy.
>
> Tinsley 1988

The initiative, which started in 1982, set up parallel systems of production and delivery projects. That is to say, it differentiated in the main between projects with a remit to *produce* materials and projects with a remit to develop systems for *delivering* the materials to the students with an appropriate support network. The results of the projects, listed in the Open Tech Directory (Partridge 1986) show an impressive, if rather patchy, provision of resources. Tinsley (1988, p193) notes that 'The early days of Open Tech brought many problems but solutions were found which have helped inform future projects and developments.'

What, then, were the achievements of the Open Tech initiative? They are probably not best expressed by totalling the products of the various projects, many of whom had enormous problems fulfilling their contracts. However, it is fair to say that the Open Tech, along with a number of other MSC initiatives aimed at different groups, changed the agenda of education. Perhaps for almost the first time, many educational institutions had to take issues of access and flexibility seriously, simply because the MSC was holding a number of the purse strings at a time of financial stringency. There were other reasons for the interest in training the existing workforce, such as the predicted decline in school leavers, but the impact of government policy was substantial, and government was (and remains) largely committed to open learning.

The Open Tech did not want the traditional institutions to stay as they were, merely adding on an open learning dimension to their existing provision. Rather, they wanted open learning to be the lever that broke the institutions open. Open learning as a term came to the fore and there was much discussion about the difference between open learning and distance learning. The importance of the distinction is discussed in the next chapter, but it is interesting to note here that the date of the change of title of the Open University sponsored journal *Teaching at a Distance* to *Open Learning* was 1986. The title change was prompted not just by the new terminology, but also because the focus of the journal had moved away from an introspective preoccupation with the Open University experience of overcoming problems of distance to include other open learning initiatives and concerns, both in the United Kingdom and abroad.

Open College

The founding of the Open College in 1987 seemed to be right on the crest of the open learning wave. Now was the time, it was said, to really take advantage of technology for communication, and the Open College was established as a national centre to broadcast TV programmes and sell supporting courses. It was focused specifically on the needs of industry.

> The Open College is an initiative that brings together broadcasters, educationalists and industry to provide vocational education and training for a mass audience. The objective is to improve the UK's economic performance.
>
> Sheila Innes, Chief Executive of the Open College (Innes 1988)

Unfortunately, such broadcasting is not cheap and the Open College ran swiftly into financial problems based on poor take-up by both individuals and corporate clients. However, the College is important in the history of open learning because it shows the perils of seduction by technology. As we have seen, the Open University was envisaged originally as relying on broadcasting and the Open College was seen as an extension of this idea into vocational education. However, media other than text make up a relatively small part of Open University production, and many Open Tech projects learned the hard way that video production is both expensive and time consuming.

Open Polytechnic

Perhaps tired of new educational institutions springing up around them, a group of polytechnics got together, in 1988, and organised the Open Polytechnic. The overt aim was to get together and produce learning materials on a consortium basis, but clearly one part of the agenda was to protect themselves from the perceived competition offered by other sources, such as the Open College. The proposal involved a substantial collaboration with a major publishing house, an idea which had been taken up on a small scale by many open learning institutions, but the Open Polytechnic intended to rely on private finance for almost all production costs. All open learning institutions have discovered that producing open learning materials is extremely expensive and, moreover, it is very difficult in most sectors of education to pass this cost on to the learner. Various packages of private and public subsidy and income from fees support other institutions but with the Open Polytechnic the balance shifted towards reliance on private funding.

European initiatives

The integration of educational systems within Europe is a goal of the Europe Commission (EC), and it is clear that the EC is committed to open learning:

> ...the Commission is fully committed to the appropriate use of open and distance learning methods as a method for delivering education and training. This commitment is also reflected by the European Parliament, for example in their endorsement of the proposals for the establishment of an European Open University, their support for programmes such as COMETT and their interest in the NEPTUNE proposals.

> Fox 1988

The move towards open learning in Europe seems to be led by the need for technology transfer and is also heavily committed to high technology methods; the COMETT programme which is building an open learning infrastructure is involved in a European satellite users network for education. Nevertheless, the Commission has identified for action some of the same problems as have been identified in the UK open learning scene:

> ...there is a critical need to raise awareness in Europe about the potential benefits and relevance of open and distance learning methods. Too often distance teaching is ignored or, at best, regarded as a second rate alternative.
> ...it is important to ensure that at all stages of the education cycle open and distance learning students are treated equitably with their counterparts who adopt more traditional routes.
> ...it is essential that whenever open and distance learning

programmes are provided, they meet the highest standards of quality and that in particular full credit recognition is given to the achievements of individuals who have studied such programmes.

Fox 1988

Assimilation or discrimination?

So where does open learning stand now? There has been both an expansion and a change in emphasis. There has been an expansion in absolute terms, since the various initiatives have brought more players into the game. However, the change in emphasis is probably even more important than the expansion. The original open learning institutions – the NEC and the Open University – were founded on the egalitarian consumerism of the 1960s; egalitarian because of the concern with access and with offering a 'second chance', and consumerism because of the emphasis on quality and standards. However, the emphasis of the 1980s and 1990s is on the needs of United Kingdom industry rather than the individual consumer of education. The success or failure of Open Tech was measured in terms of the impact on British industry and the enthusiasm of British industrialists. And to a degree these industrialists were enthusiastic about the potential of open learning to train the workforce, although, as McNay (1988) points out, they also said that open learning saved them money. The importance of personal liberation for the learner was not a key component of the evaluation of Open Tech, but there was a recognition that open learning transferred some power to the individual learner. If nothing else, it allowed her to improve her skills and thus have more resources to trade with her employer. But, as McNay again reminds us, this is only true if the skills which she has learnt are generic, and not specific to the post or firm she is in.

Thus, there is now a tension in open learning between the ideals of egalitarian consumerism and the objectives of industry driven training. This tension is particularly uncomfortable because, to an extent, open learning remains marginalised; it exists apart from the mainstream of education. However, there is some indication that the marginalisation of open learning is coming to an end. This is mainly due to changes within education as a whole which favour the development of open learning or, more accurately, remove some of the constraints which inhibited open learning. Changes include the increased use of open learning in schools as part of a philosophy of student-centred learning, the changing role and philosophy of accrediting agencies, and the growth of the full-cost sector in higher education. Of the accrediting agencies, the Business and Technical Education Council (BTEC) has always looked favourably on open learning and seen it fitting in with its modular schemes, and the Council for National Academic Awards (CNAA) has, under the Credit Accumulation and Transfer Scheme

(CATS), looked increasingly favourably at open learning within modular courses. It is the integration of open learning with the mainstream of accreditation which will, in my view, earn open learning a key role in adult education.

So, has open learning grown up? It is impossible to be sure about the *age* of open learning because we have no 'full lifetime' to compare it too. However, it does seem to have changed its gender stereotype. In the past it was intended to appeal to the disabled of society – women, people with physical disabilities, and the poor, although the record of attracting these groups was sometimes disappointing. Today, however, open learning has a much more robust 'macho' image. 'Real men do it openly' would make a good T-shirt slogan. But, of course, nursing is not full of men but of women, many of them disadvantaged in multiple ways: so what of open learning in nursing?

Open learning in nursing

The Open Tech initiative brought open learning firmly into nursing education, but the learning packages offered through that programme were not the first to be made specifically for nurses. In the early 1980s the Open University had been approached with the idea of making materials to help nurses master the (then new) nursing process. The outcome was a pack: *P553 A Systematic Approach to Nursing Care* (Open University 1984) which is the most widely used learning package within nursing. Sales figures quoted by the Open University indicate total sales between the launch in 1984 and the end of 1988 in excess of 20,000, and it has been estimated that real usage increases that figure by a factor of 3 (Liddiard 1989).

However, the adoption of *P553* by nurse educators should not be equated with the introduction of open learning. It was seen in general as a specific answer to a specific problem, as a 'one-off' tool which would not disrupt or alter the way in which conventional teaching went on. There is no evidence that it was seen as a portent of a revolution – and indeed it wasn't. The Open University failed to follow up the success of that pack with any other pack specifically for nurses, although nurses were obviously included in the potential audience for their other courses and many nurses were attempting to increase their academic qualifications through the undergraduate programme. The pool of expertise which was built up during the production of the course was dissipated and the initiative passed to the Open Tech.

As the Open Tech initiative was intended to update workers in British industry in new technical expertise, it is not quite clear how the inclusion of nurses – experts in 'people work' rather than high tech industry – came to be included. However, they secured not one but two contracts, out of a total of about 140. The larger of the two projects was based at South Bank Polytechnic, which already had a large nursing department. The second project was based at Barnet College, which was already heavily involved in Flexistudy, in collaboration with Central Manchester College.

Distance Learning Centre

The project at South Bank Polytechnic was based, not in the nursing department, but with other open learning projects in the continuing education department and took the modest title of Distance Learning Centre (DLC). The intent was to take advantage of economies of scale for the production and distribution facilities. The emphasis was very much on the use of information technology in all stages of the process and there was heavy investment in both hardware and software. This approach could be said to follow the Open University example of large scale production, although the scale of the enterprise at South Bank Polytechnic was much smaller. The project had the advantage of not being constrained by working practices agreed in the 1960s (which had inhibited the introduction of new technology at the Open University).

The original contract was to produce materials to support the Diploma in Nursing but there was very swift negotiation to move some production capacity to more financially viable products. These issues are explored more closely in the account of the setting up of the DLC in Chapter 4. In general the project was established very much along the lines pioneered by the Open University, probably because the first director of the DLC had come from the Open University. In particular, it was assumed from the first that the centre would be primarily a teaching centre serving students rather than a publishing centre dealing with sales. It must also be said that members of the Open University were very willing to help struggling Open Tech projects with advice on all aspects of production and distribution and most staff recruited to the DLC explored Open University models before evolving their own systems.

Continuing Nurse Education

The project based at Barnet College followed a different set of precedents. The first director had worked extensively with Flexistudy materials, and the format for the production of materials which they eventually adopted looked much like NEC materials. The production and distribution centre was initially based at Central Manchester College, again to some extent to take advantage of economies of scale, but it was modelled more closely on a small printer or a small college publishing facility, rather than the Open University.

Although funded as projects, both the DLC and Continuing Nurse Education (CNE) very rapidly began to plan for a longer life. It was assumed that the desirable outcome was the establishment of permanent centres of open learning – in the case of the DLC dealing both with production and delivery to students – serving nursing and health care. The first, and most important issue, was of course finance. Both projects embarked on ambitious programmes of production but realised that the market existed only as a potential. Nobody was clamouring for open learning materials, although a number of people supported the idea. The most supportive nurse tutors were almost invariably those who had themselves obtained a degree through the Open University. They therefore began to liaise with the professional and statutory bodies to explore the place of open learning. Immediately the problem was obvious: the place of open learning is dependent on decisions about the structure and philosophy of pre- and post-registration education. Between 1984 and 1986, when the projects most needed to plan with some certainty about what would be acceptable to nurses, there was increasing uncertainty about nurse education.

The employers' initiative

It has always been generally recognised that, as an 'industry', the National Health Service had no overall strategy on education and training which included all the different occupations, and the Health Pickup scheme was part of a large strategy to deal with training needs. It was launched in the mid-1980s by the Department of Education and Science (DES) and the National Health Service Training Authority (NHSTA) with great enthusiasm but perhaps less understanding of what it could or should do – and who should do it. The objectives were to produce open learning materials for all sectors of nursing and for the professions allied to medicine. The programme of work which was eventually agreed consisted of a needs analysis followed by the production of a number of open learning modules on various topics. The first six were:

- the role of the professional in charge
- setting objectives and standards for care
- assessing needs and priorities
- managing the caseload and time
- helping staff learn through experience
- working with other professions

The basic idea was to have a complete range of learning packs to cover the whole range of service training needs with the exception of clinical training and management training. In the words of the NHSTA it 'is not intended to replace existing training initiatives. It offers an additional resource to supplement and support existing activity.'

Management training is covered by the management training syllabus and open learning project (MESOL). The foundation course, which is designed to meet the needs of those moving into management for the first time was commissioned in 1988 and is being jointly developed by the Open University and the Institute of Health Services Management (IHSM). The whole scheme is based on the accumulation and transfer of credits towards both Open University and IHSM qualifications, and hopefully other managerial and professional qualifications. Students will be supported by tutors and workplace mentors.

Neither of these initiatives, of course, deal with clinical education which is assumed, in public at least, to be the business of the appropriate professional bodies. But of course it is not easy to say where clinical education begins and ends, and the list of topics covered by Health Pickup would certainly be covered within many nursing courses. Similarly, management issues could be said to be central to all good nursing practice. So what is happening within the professions?

The professional initiative

Both the DLC and the CNE saw the importance of involving the National Boards and the United Kingdom Central Council (UKCC) in their planning, and formal links were made through the steering groups and informal ones through workshops and discussions at various levels. However, the development of the open learning projects came at a time when the statutory bodies were overwhelmingly concerned with Project 2000 and close involvement in other issues, particularly in continuing education, was resisted. Nevertheless, the statutory bodies did show an interest in open learning in a number of ways. The English National Board (ENB) established an Open Learning Working Group as a sub-group to the Continuing Education Committee of the Board with the remit: 'To consider the potential of open learning for nursing, midwifery and health visiting education and to advise the Continuing Education Committee of the Board'. Part of the work of the Group involved producing criteria for the approval of open learning courses, and indeed the Board was approving courses with a substantial open learning component, such as the mixed mode course ENB 870 described in Chapter 12. The ENB also began to produce its own open learning packs for particular markets which it had identified. The National Board for Scotland was also interested in the potential of open learning and collaborated with the innovative programme established in the Highland Health Board which is described in Chapter 15. The Welsh National Board has had a very positive approach to open learning, and has good links with the Open University Regional Office in Cardiff. It intends to use open learning where appropriate to promote access to the new framework for professional practice.

However, it was apparent to many open learning enthusiasts that the breakthrough in support for open learning would come with mandatory periodic updating. This would ensure that funds for continuing education – whether from public or private sources – would dramatically increase but the constraints on releasing staff for education would remain. The obvious solution would be open learning. The first two stages of that development – the work on the conversion course and the return to practice courses both specifically mentioned open learning routes. However, the primary motivation for the promotion of open learning seems to have been the logistical problems of providing continuing education to the nursing workforce. The ideas of egalitarianism and consumerism which inspired the foundation of the NEC and the Open University have been largely absent from the discussion in nursing. In this, the introduction of open learning in nursing follows the trend of other vocational learning.

The Department of Health

The Department of Health was interested in open learning in the context of its concern with continuing education for the nursing workforce, and as their funded research project on continuing education came to an end (Rogers and Lawrence 1987) they supported a new initiative to look at the role of open learning in nurse education. Interestingly, the original initiative for the project had come from the DLC, which saw its brief as promoting research into open learning in general rather than just into its own materials and courses.

However, it was at the end of the 1980s that the whole importance of open learning in nurse education changed gear. A major investment by the Department of Health enabled work on open learning in the context of continuing education for nurses to move forward on a number of fronts. A tripartite programme of projects was established looking at:

- the philosophy of continuing education
- the promotion of open learning in schools of nursing via collaborative ventures, helping the tutors assess their role, etc.
- an accreditation scheme, involving credits for experience, courses and open learning, rather along the lines of the CNAA Credit Accumulation and Transfer Scheme (CATS).

Piggy in the middle

Both the statutory bodies for nursing and the employer's training agency – the NHSTA – are therefore heavily committed to open learning. There is a potential division of responsibility between clinical issues, which belong to the profession, and management and occupational issues, which belong to the NHSTA. The problem, of course, is that it is difficult to break an individual's training needs down into the two categories, although it is important to recognise the inherent tension between them. For vocational training in nursing, therefore, open learning becomes embroiled in the politics of occupational control and professional aspirations. The institutional division, however, is not the same as in other areas of open learning. For example, the DLC and the CNE, which were Open Tech projects, are allied more firmly with the professional interests than with the managers of the service. The professional 'voice' has always been overwhelmingly represented on the steering groups, indeed the CNE is embedded in the Royal College of Nursing, and they have worked closely with the National Boards. While approaches were made to both the DLC and CNE projects by Health Pickup, in the event, there was no collaboration or integration of materials or programmes on the first phase of Health Pickup.

While the open learning scene is now a busy one, therefore, it is by no means a coordinated one and the individual nurse and the nurse teacher are to some extent caught in the middle. While more materials are being offered to them they have very little guidance on how to sensibly use the materials to fulfil their objectives. Few teachers or nurses have been trained to cope with the demands of open learning which is still being introduced within conventional institutions and structures. And the materials are themselves offering mixed messages: some are asking the nurse to improve her educational abilities and think creatively; others are concerned to help her to grasp some of the technical problems of being a cog in a big machine. A reaction along the lines of 'a plague on both your houses' would be understandable.

The nurse teachers have in general been slow to become involved in open learning, although there are a number of schools which have been very enthusiastic, perhaps because the teachers most interested in principles of openness in education more often expressed it through work with experiential learning, learning contracts, etc. They actively rejected open learning because they felt that it would remove the face-to-face communication which for them is at the heart of teaching and provides much of their job satisfaction. Nevertheless, there has been sufficient interest for many innovative schemes to get off the ground, as will be seen in later chapters, but it is probably true to say that open learning is most usually seen as a solution to a specific problem rather than a fundamental challenge to the way we currently do things – it remains marginalised in all but a handful of districts.

What of the future?

The future of open learning in nursing, of course, depends on a number of things other than its efficiency and efficacy. It depends how it fits in with the plans and programmes of the various bodies which are competing for the soul of nurse education – the NHSTA, the national boards, the UKCC, the Department of Health and the Department of Education and Science. Each of the interested parties will see the purpose of open learning differently and therefore define and operationalise it differently. These definitions and projects will draw, implicitly or explicitly, on the range of precedents from outside the health care sector and the literature on open learning. Regrettably they may look only for simple solutions and avoid some of the lessons to be learnt. What then are the definitions of open learning which are in general use; how is the discussion about open learning in general progressing? The next chapter will look more closely at this issue.

References

Ellwood C 1976 *Adult Learning Today: a New Role for the Universities?* Sage

Fox N H M 1988 The EC's Education Policies and programmes: the COMETT Programme, paper presented to the 14th World Conference on Distance Education, Oslo 9-16 August, 1988.

Innes S 1988 The Open College: a personal view. In Paine N (ed) 1988 *Open Learning in Transition*. National Extension College

Jenkins J and Perraton H 1980 *The Invisible College NEC 1963-1979* IEC Broadsheets on Distance Learning No 15. International Extension College

Liddiard P 1989 Personal communication

McNay I 1988 Open learning: a jarring note. In Paine N (ed) 1988 *Open Learning in Transition*. National Extension College

Open University 1984 *P553 A Systematic Approach to Nursing Care: an Introduction* The Open University Press

OU 1988 *Open Learning* (DO5 Part B/E86-, Module 2, Professional Studies in Post-compulsory Education). The Open University Press

Paine N (ed) 1988 *Open Learning in Transition*. National Extension College

Partridge L (ed) 1986 *Open Tech Directory*. National Extension College/Manpower Services Commission

Perry W 1976 *Open University*. The Open University Press

Rogers J and Lawrence J 1987 *Continuing Professional Education for Qualified Nurses, Midwives and Health Visitors.* Ashdale Press and Austen Cornish Publishers

Tinsley D 1988 Facing the future: the role of the Training Commission in support of open learning. In Paine N (ed) 1988 *Open Learning in Transition.* National Extension College

2 Open learning: definitions and debates

Kate Robinson

Open learning – whatever it is – is a highly problematic, contested terrain.
Lentell 1989

The historical account of the growth of open learning in the previous chapter looked at a number of institutional themes which are generally thought of as coming under the 'open learning' umbrella. However, it is now time to consider what holds these disparate institutions together; to ask whether there is an identifiable philosophy or criteria which all those involved in these institutions would recognise and be happy to accept as a description of their activity. It is important not to detach concepts from the particular institutional contexts and social relationships in which they are embedded, and all the accounts of open learning in subsequent sections of the book deal with specific courses and programmes. However, it is also important to have one place in the book where the underlying issues and themes can be spelt out and untangled from their origins. So, although I would not want to dissent from Helen Lendell's statement which opened this chapter, I do want to try to construct a guide to the terrain to lead you through some of the discussions and definitions about the nature of open learning which have grown up in parallel with practical developments.

The books on open learning are riddled with attempts to define *open learning* and to distinguish it from *distance learning*, and often the former is seen as the umbrella term, with distance learning as a subset. However, a number of authors (*see*, for example, Keegan 1986 and Rumble 1989) have argued very persuasively that this is inappropriate, and may lead to important misunderstandings. The following discussion, therefore, looks at distance learning and open learning separately, before examining the possibility of a useful synthesis.

Distance learning

Although *distance learning* is the commonly used term, Keegan (1986) has argued that *distance education* is more appropriate because it can subsume both distance *learning* and distance *teaching*, that is, the two aspects which are necessary for a complete educational experience. The distinction can be important because it helps to distinguish the kinds of formal systems that teachers are most concerned about from the sort of informal learning that goes on every time someone opens a book.

Distance education is not, of course, a phenomena confined to the United Kingdom, although the Open University is a major international focal point for the development of distance teaching, and definitions cannot therefore be based solely on UK experience. However, after a comprehensive examination of educational systems throughout the world, Keegan proposes the following definition :

Distance education is a form of education characterised by

- the quasi-permanent separation of teacher and learner throughout the length of the learning process; this distinguishes it from conventional face-to-face education.
- The influence of an educational organisation both in the planning and preparation of learning materials and in the provision of student support services; this distinguishes it from private study and teach-yourself programmes.
- the use of technical media; print, audio, video or computer, to unite teacher and learner and carry the content of the course.
- the provision of two-way communication so that the student may benefit from or even initiate dialogue; this distinguishes it from other uses of technology in education.
- the quasi-permanent absence of the learning group throughout the length of the learning process so that people are usually taught as individuals and not in groups, with the possibility of occasional meetings for both didactic and socialisation purposes.

Keegan 1986

The most important of these criteria is the first; whatever else it might be, distance education is a non-contiguous learning situation, that is, the teacher and learner are separated in time and space. This contrasts with the contiguous learning situation of conventional education. The distance created by the lack of contiguity between teacher and learner is bridged by the use of various technologies - print, telephone, etc. Two further elements have been proposed by Keegan; both are controversial but neither are essential criteria; he categorises them rather as elements necessarily attached to distance education. The first element, which he attributes to Peters (1965), is the *industrialisation* of the process of teaching concomitant with the use of media and of telecommunications. In its simplest form one can readily see that a distance teaching institution like the Open University is involved in the mass production of teaching materials for mass consumption by students. One can also argue that the separation of the producer and the consumer, which is a key feature of distance education, is characteristic of industrial systems.

The second element is what Keegan calls the *privatisation* of the learner. This is important because it is a definition of the elements of the system which offer independence, autonomy and freedom to the learner. Keegan argues that the concept of independence does not reflect the realities of systems in which the learners' path is clearly laid down and circumscribed by pre-set syllabi and assessments. This is a topic which we will return to later in our discussion of open learning. Before we leave the topic of distance education, it is worth pointing out what it excludes, which is the use of learning materials within conventional classroom settings or for private study.

What emerges from the definitions given above that the term *distance* describes a *method* or *means* of teaching rather than any philosophy or ideology of learning. Distance teaching, in this sense, grew up to provide alternative learning opportunities for those who could not attend conventional courses. It can be thought of as 'second-best' or a 'route of last resort' because it struggles to overcome the problems created by the distance between teacher and learner; contiguity remains, in this view, the ideal teaching situation (*see,* for example, the rationale for the National Extension College in Chapter 1). The advantages of distance education lie very much in the economies of scale, which allow a large number of learners to be serviced at a low unit cost, and of privatisation, which allows the learner to remain within other social contexts even while becoming a student at an educational institution. We can also begin to see from the references to the Open University, why there is confusion about the terms 'open' and 'distance'; The Open University was originally envisaged as the University of the Air, a title which drew attention to the use of media in the teaching process (although in practice the system depends on print rather than broadcasting), however the title of 'Open' was eventually adopted to emphasise the recruitment policy which was (and is) to offer courses to people without conventional university entrance qualifications. The issue of recruitment is not encompassed within the definition of distance education offered by Keegan, and from which therefore it could be argued that it is not an essential part of the institution. However, it does mean that the principle distance teaching institution in the UK is connected to open learning via its title; it remains to be seen whether there are other more important connections.

B

Open learning

What then is open learning? Openness is popularly construed as the removal of barriers which stand between the learner and education: 'There is no universally agreed definition of open learning. The essential idea, however, is that of opening up new opportunities for people to learn.' (MSC 1988). The opposite of 'open' is of course 'closed', but Lewis and Spencer (1986) have developed the idea of openness as a continuum and suggest that each aspect of learner choice can be defined as being somewhere along a continuum from open to closed. The relevant aspects of learner choice are defined as:

- *whether* or not to learn
- *what* to learn
- *how* to learn (methods, media, routes)
- *where* to learn (the place of learning)
- *when* to learn (start and finish, pace)
- *who* to turn to for help (tutors? trainers? friends? colleagues?)
- *how* to get learning assessed (and the nature of the feedback provided)
- *what* to do *next* (other courses? career direction?)

This sort of approach constructs openness as a multidimensional concept and other definitions will usually offer some selection from the list above depending on the context of the discussion. Rumble (1989) has examined the various criteria found in the literature and proposes a five-fold category system to encompass the various selections:

- access-related criteria
- criteria related to place and pace of study
- criteria related to means
- criteria related to support services.
- criteria related to the structure of the programme in respect of content and assessment

I will look briefly at each of these in turn.

Access
These criteria are concerned with characteristics of the learner which would normally prevent them being allowed to join a course. It includes, for example, lack of appropriate academic or vocational qualifications, inappropriate age, lack of adequate financial support, and the inability to attend a class because of physical handicap or social circumstances, such as being in prison.

Place and pace
Learners may want to choose when and where to study and in this context, openness would indicate, for example, no fixed attendance times and no start date or completion date. Courses would be organised on a 'roll-on, roll-off' basis with the learner dictating the intervening timetable. Where equipment was necessary for the completion of the course this should either be offered to each learner or provided in a group facility with very generous times for access.

Means
If a learner can choose the means of study then the implication is that a variety of parallel methods of delivery, such as text, audio-tape, interactive video, etc. must be available, with a redundancy factor built in. In other words, the learner could choose from a selection of methods and need not use them all.

Support services
Support services, which are usually provided by teachers, peers, and others, may be provided in a variety of forms in a variety of places. They may be proactively offered to the learner or they may require activating by learner action.

Content and assessment
These criteria centre around the question, 'How far can the learner define their own learning aims and assess whether they have been met?'. As a minimum, a syllabus may offer a choice of topics which relate to the learner's interests and allow learners with existing knowledge to avoid repeating subjects, but the opportunities for learner definition of content may go further to perhaps an individual learning contract for each learner. Again as a minimum the learner may be able to choose from a menu of assessment methods, or she may simply be able to define when her learning needs have been satisfactorily met.

Any definition of openness may invoke one or more of these sets of criteria or define the elements of a criteria differently, as can be seen from this brief selection of definitions:

> Open Learning: arrangements to enable people to learn at the time, place and pace which satisfies their circumstances and requirements. The emphasis is on opening up opportunities by overcoming barriers that result from geographical isolation, personal or work commitments or conventional course structures which have often prevented people from gaining access to the training they need.

> MSC 1984 (cited in Lewis 1986)

'Open Learning' is a term used to describe courses flexibly designed to meet individual requirements. It is often applied to provision which tries to remove barriers that prevent attendances at more traditional courses, but it also suggests a learner-centred philosophy. Open learning courses may be offered in a learning centre of some kind or more of the activity may be carried out away from such a centre (eg at home). In nearly every case specially prepared or adapted materials are necessary.

Lewis and Spencer 1986

...open learning is an attempt to break down the traditional barriers to training such as pre-qualification, age, geographical location, availability, scheduling, learning style and cost.

Cooper 1987 cited in Fricker 1988

Open learning - a term used to describe education and training schemes designed to meet the varied requirements of individuals - for example as to what, where, when and how they learn. This freedom is achieved by providing carefully planned, flexible learning packages.

Marson undated

Open and distance: opposites or bedfellows?

Having explored the definitions of distance education and open learning, we are now in a position to define their relationship with each other. Escotet clearly sees a sharp distinction between the two concepts :

Open education is particularly characterised by the removal of restrictions, exclusions and privileges; by the accreditation of students' previous experiences; by the flexibility of the management of the time variable; and by substantial changes in the traditional relationship between professors and students. *On the other hand*, distance education is a modality which permits the delivery of a group of didactic media without the necessity of regular class participation, where the individual is responsible for his own learning.

Escotet 1983 cited in Keegan 1986 (My emphasis)

However, others see the distinction as more apparent than real:

> Open learning is a phrase with a positive ring to it. It is one of a family of terms all of which stress to varying degrees the centrality of learner choice (cf 'learner-directed training', 'self-study', 'independent learning'), the use of materials (cf 'packaged training', 'resource-based learning') and of flexible delivery methods (cf 'flexistudy, 'distance learning', 'computer-based training').
>
> Lewis 1986

> Distance learning is but one variant of open learning...
>
> Thorpe and Grugeon 1987

The source of the difficulty in distinguishing between the two concepts lies in the breadth of the definitions of open learning, a concept which has grown to encompass almost all educational activity other than the most traditional of work in the classroom. It seems to me that the collection of criteria which has been assembled by the advocates of open learning encompasses components which are not of equal value or weight and which need to be evaluated rather than simply listed. It may be that some of the criteria are more related to the idea of distance education and that this generates some of the confusion between the two terms. The one thing we can say about the criteria, therefore, is that they are not homogeneous.

The heterogeneity of the criteria

Unlike the definition of distance education, where the idea of non-contiguity was seen to be central to the issue, there is very little agreement in the literature about which criteria might be essential to a definition of open. Lewis, using the 'open-closed continuum' model, suggests:

> This model may be used to analyse any open learning schemes. The most familiar open learning system, the Open University undergraduate programme, is a good example to start with. This is very open on WHO? and WHY?; moderately open on WHERE?; both open and closed on WHAT? and HOW?; and finally very closed on WHEN?
>
> Lewis 1986

Lewis makes no conceptual distinction between the categories of who, why, where, what, how and when. Following this process it would be possible to accept within the 'open' umbrella systems which had diametrically opposed characteristics. For example, unlike the analysis of the Open University above, they might be very closed on 'who' and 'why' and very open on 'when'; and indeed, as we shall see later, an open learning system in nursing is likely to have great difficulties with the category of 'who'. Do these differences matter? I want to argue that they do because the implications of adopting the various criteria are very different and will lead both to different structures but also to different types of experience for the learner.

To say that the learner may study at a place and time of her own convenience, for example, requires that the teacher assembles some learning materials for the learner and abandons classroom teaching. In a sophisticated system, the materials would be well packaged, possibly multi-media, the learner would be offered support of some kind, such as telephone tutorials, and there would be a complex record system, probably computer based. However, the essential relationship between the teacher and learner is not explicitly altered.

Consider, on the other hand, the implications of changing the content and assessment criteria to enhance the learner's ability to:

> ... define his or her own learning objectives, determine the content which he or she should study, negotiate the provision of services to help him or her master the syllabus, and construct and agree the method of assessment to be used.

> Rumble 1989

This clearly proposes a complete realignment of the relationship between teacher and learner and the cession of power from the former to the latter in a dramatic fashion. The learner takes control of her situation and the teacher's role moves significantly towards facilitation of learning rather than the transmission of information. Openness in this context means 'learner-centred' *and* 'learner-controlled'.

As the differences between the criteria are so important it seems useful to distinguish between issues of *open access* - the removal of barriers - and *open pedagogy* [1]- the realignment of control. This distinction can help to explain the confusion between open and distance learning in that the characteristics of open access are very similar to the characteristics of a distance learning system, For example, both will probably provide learning packages to enable the learner to study at a time and place of her choosing, both may be of use to learners who are unable to attend conventional courses. The similarity arises because non-contiguity is a successful solution to many of the problems of providing access to courses. However, a distance learning course may not have any of the characteristics of open pedagogy; it may be 'closed' in the sense of being teacher-centred.

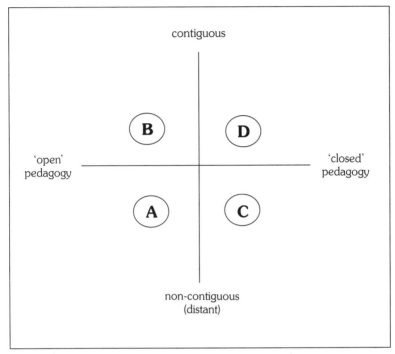

Figure 2.1   Interactivity between open and distance learning

Constructing a matrix

While the concept of open access remains within the concept of openness, it is impossible to clearly distinguish between open learning and distance learning. However, using the concept of open pedagogy we can construct a matrix to see how they might interact (Figure 2.1). Clearly open pedagogy can be applied to both contiguous and non-contiguous systems. A distance system could be open, but it may not be; an open system could be non-contiguous, or it may not.

However, I want to argue that a system which may be called 'open' but which is concerned only with criteria of pace, place and time - the three criteria often quoted in connection with the Open Tech programme - may lie in quadrant C; those which emphasised learner control but did not set it in a context of learning materials would lie in quadrant B, and those which emphasised both learner-centredness and set it within a framework of support structures available at a distance would lie in quadrant A. This is, of course, an oversimplification, and each quadrant in itself contains multiple possibilities of emphasis between the two indices. This matrix also indicates why there has been antagonism towards open learning within nursing from those who one might have supposed would have been inclined to support it. Protagonists of independent learning may have identified open learning with a closed pedagogy, even though access was open, and placed it correctly in quadrant C, where it appears diametrically opposed with their own position in quadrant B. Because those keen on promoting an open pedagogy, also within a non-contiguous system, use the same label extensive dialogue would have to take place before common interests could be identified. Such dialogue has not really started within nursing.

Some of the confusion has arisen because education in general has been under pressure, because of the new emphases on individual learning, to move towards openness. Within adult education, where substantial numbers of learners are already in non-contiguous systems such as the Open University, there has been movement from C to A. However, because of the potential opportunities for learner-centredness which non-contiguity offers, there has also been movement from D to A. And, just to ensure that the waters are thoroughly muddied, there has been a movement from D to C, mainly within the industrial training sector, on the ground that non-contiguity is a very efficient and effective way of delivering standardised training to a scattered workforce.

These movements can be located within specific insitutions and educational sectors. For example, the move from a closed/contiguous to a closed/non-contiguous system was characteristic of much, although not all, of the Open Tech programme. The Open College is similarly concerned with the logistics of training rather than any learner-centred definition of openness. And a case could be made that the Open Polytechnic is also concerned with the logistics of reaching a wider market rather than pedagogy. However, there may be differences even within one institution; the Open University, for example, contains sectors which emphasise the importance of maintaining control despite the distance separating learner and teacher, although other sectors, particularly in the continuing education programme, are more interested in the educational opportunities afforded by distance. Nevertheless, despite the distinctions being made here, the fact remains that institutions and programmes which have very little in common pedagogically will continue to claim the title 'open learning' simply because currently a certain amount of 'kudos' and respectability adheres to it - or to put it rather more crudely, open learning is the 'flavour of the month'.

The matrix biases

I have argued that all four quadrants of the matrix can potentially be filled, but is this likely to occur in practice? Does the movement to teaching at a distance create the conditions in which an open pedagogy always flourishes? Similarly does an open pedagogy always involve an element of distance and a reliance on the learning materials which are characteristic of distance systems?

The idea that an open pedagogy generates the use of learning materials is the easier of the two questions to answer; I find it difficult to see how control can be exercised by a learner without breaking the dependence on contiguity, and to break this dependence without providing some substance to replace some of the functions of the teacher simply abdicates the teacher's role in education. Once part of the syllabus is encapsulated in a permanent medium, such as audiotape or text, then the learner can use it in a way that they cannot use a teacher. Some obvious examples of the problems with the conventional role of teachers are that they are not available 24 hours a day, they are not entirely happy with repeating material, running it the other way, going back to what they said ten minutes ago, or checking if they are using terms entirely consistently by rerunning their whole year's input. In contrast, all these things are perfectly possible with the well designed open learning package. Obviously I am aware that a number of teachers in contiguous educational situations, including myself, like to believe that we are 'open', but I suspect that we underestimate the power of our role and mistake the sharing of power with 'user-friendliness'.

The question of whether distance systems have an automatic bias towards openness is more complex. Much of the technology used, particularly printed text, allows for a change in the balance of power between teacher and learner. Because the primary vehicle for teaching is in the hands of the learner she has a number of freedoms beyond the obvious ones of being able to learn where and when she wants. She can, for instance, use the text in a non-linear fashion to construct a more meaningful learning experience. The degree of freedom is to some extent dependent on the technology involved. Broadcasting, for example, constrains both where and when learning can take place; however, in contrast, the introduction of the home video recorder allows students to record broadcasts and to watch them whenever and how often they like and not just when they are 'programmed' in.

However, the alternative argument can be put:

> There can be no doubt that the control of the curriculum and the isolation of the student body which are features of distance education make distance education a ready vehicle for

totalitarian control of education.

Rumble 1989

Once the syllabus has been enshrined in materials then it tends to be unavailable for negotiation, and there may well be a tendency to concentrate on the materials aspect of the system rather than the learner support. This is partly because of the industrial nature of the production process which squeezes out other concerns, but also because the materials are in the public domain, and will therefore be examined by the author's peers, while the support of the individual learner will not. In theory the tutor within the support system will mediate the effects of the materials. Sewart (1988) and Tait (1988), writing of the Open University, argue that tuition and counselling within the support system:

> ...have an essential role in individualising mass produced course materials and encouraging students to make sense of knowledge and information on their own terms. Tuition and counselling oppose the potential of distance education for totalitarian practice where a monopoly on what is allowed as knowledge can be enshrined in the course units.

Tait 1988

However, this view seems to me to underestimate the importance of the assessment system over which even the tutors may have little control, and the role of the tutor could be described as persuading the students to accept the version of events proposed by the authors of the course units in order that they may pass the examination which is almost certainly set by some of the authors.

However, the main system for controlling learners within distance teaching systems is the assessment system which prescribes how much the learners should have learned of the given material by a certain date. Using the Open University again as an example, the assessment schemes on the majority of their courses constrain the student within fairly tight timetables. The course U205 *Health and Disease*, for example, has seven assignments spread throughout their academic year – from January to November – with fixed submission dates (the usual term 'cut-off dates' conveys the message very well) and a final examination.

What does an open learning system look like?

What does it mean to operationalise this troublesome concept of open learning; what does the practice which gives rise to the theory, look like? Within the previous discussion I have been trading on a distinction between the production of learning materials and the support of learning which needs some expansion. However, in order to describe an open learning system we need to move away from the complexities of the debate in the previous sections and clarify what will 'count', at least for the purposes of this chapter, as open learning. Having distinguished the various issues and concepts, one from another, it does not follow that I necessarily want to enforce them on the world of practice as stipulated definitions. Rather, as I indicated in the last chapter, I am going to use open learning as the umbrella term here, not because it has any academic currency, but partly in the interests of brevity and partly because it reflects current usage within the field of open and distance learning. And open learning, as we have seen, within its broadest definition could encompass almost anything. So the following description will relate to the majority of courses or programmes which might call themselves, open learning, that is, they are non-contiguous systems based on learning materials of one sort or another, where the learner is supported to various degrees by teachers who are aware of the importance of learner-centredness, although the degree of pedagogic control ceded to the learner will vary enormously.

Such a system needs to carry out three primary functions:

- creation of materials
- provision of support to the learner
- administration and management of the system(s)

and may therefore be split into three subsystems: production, delivery, and administration.

One way of categorising open learning systems is based on the extent to which these functions are brought together within one organisation or divided up between several. For example, producers of materials may be concerned only with the creation process, and deliverers only with delivering the materials to the students and providing support. (Both functions inevitably involving a complex administration system.) Such a division of responsibility was encouraged by the Open Tech which saw the delivery function as generic, rather than subject specific, and tended to organise delivery projects geographically. Nevertheless, many organisations perform both functions: the Open University, for example, creates almost all the materials which it uses and operates a complex regional structure to support the students. Similarly, the Distance Learning Centre both produces the materials for, and tutors, the Diploma in Nursing course (this course is described further in Chapter 11). However, the materials produced by both institutions are also available for sale and may also, therefore, be incorporated into other delivery systems controlled by other institutions.

The partition of functions obviously makes coordination and collaboration between the different systems a central issue, and this can apply even when all the functions are within one organisation. Within the Open University, for example, there is a tension between the central core of staff involved with production and those within the regional organisation who are involved with support (Perry 1976). Tension between different pedagogical aspirations is particularly problematic as it results in learners getting 'mixed messages' about their role, and tutors, as indicated above, have to be alert to the dangers of encouraging learner autonomy within a 'closed' syllabus and assessment system. The controlling influence within the system is very often with the production part of the trilogy, simply because this comes sequentially first and therefore sets the parameters for the learner support which follows. This can be overcome, as in the Open University, by inviting support staff into production teams. Where the systems are split between institutions greater effort needs to be made to involve the potential consumers. Alternatively the materials can be produced in very flexible formats which lend themselves to different uses and degrees of support.

The following chapter will offer an overview of production, but very briefly it involves the construction of a curriculum, deciding on appropriate media, and the translation of the curriculum into materials - audio-tape, text, video-tape or whatever, which are designed to provide, in conjunction with the learner's activities, the required learning experience. Because the learner is not present to provide feedback, the draft materials are usually tested by groups of 'typical' learners; and a further check is usually provided by experts in the relevant field. A teacher in this situation therefore spends time in drafting curricula and materials for future use by students she may never see. Because of the production aspects, the work of the teacher has to fit into a complex network of editors, transformers, designers and printers and the financial consequences of any problems with the teaching, ie the production of materials will be magnified many times beyond what could be expected in a similar classroom situation.

The support or delivery system will involve getting the materials to the learners - a difficult job if large numbers are involved - and helping the learner to maximise her learning experience by offering individual or group tuition, 'trouble-shooting', and assessment - the exact mix will depend on the system. A major part of the role will involve helping the learner choose the right course or module. Again these issues will be expanded in a later chapter (Chapter 9).

What of the learner in an open learning system? From the discussion above it is clear that the learner could be engaged in any number of activities and perhaps we can only be definite about saying that they are unlikely to be sitting in a lecture (although the Open University summer schools do offer lectures!). In general, however, they are likely to be working through a learning package of some kind either at home or in the workplace and according to their own work schedule. Ideally they will have a source of support available at short notice either in person or at the end of a telephone.

Vocational open learning

The growth of open learning in the context of vocational education has highlighted the tension between open access and open pedagogy. And to a degree the debate has centred on vocational issues because of the importance of the Open Tech programme. The aims of the programme were explicitly concerned with providing the workforce with industrially useful competence rather than competencies related to life in more general terms. In relation to the old dichotomy, it was about training rather than education. Access was a central issue because it was acknowledged that the workforce needed to be trained *as it worked* and so the open access aspects of open learning were seized as an essential part of the process. The other key word for the programme was relevance, but of course this begs the question of 'relevant to whom?' Just who, in vocational open learning, is the consumer?

Who is the consumer?

Because open learning is explicitly concerned with both the relationship between the learner and the teacher and the *control* of learning, the definition of the consumer is a vital one. There is a tripartite relationship between the teacher, the learner and the employer. In practice, there has been a fourth player in the game; because of the provision of subsidy for the development of open learning: 'the backers of the Open Learning show have been the government' (Manpower Policy and Practice 1986). It has been argued that the result of this partnership has been instrumental training which contradicts almost all aspects of openness contained in definitions except for the logistical emphasis on open access. And it could be argued that this, far from opening up opportunities, has simply increased the privatisation of training and placed more responsibility on the consumer who may not have a home situation conducive to study (Hirst 1986).

Nurse education - is openness possible?

So, is open learning a practical possibility within nurse education? Clearly there are some criteria which could not be applied in nurse education; the access-related criteria are particularly problematic.

There has been considerable discussion within the context of Project 2000 about the possibility of removing entrance criteria for pre-registration training, although in the end considerable barriers to entry remain, but clearly post-registration training is fundamentally based on the idea that entrants have particular competencies. The possibility of training as a nurse despite an inability to leave one's environment is also self-evidently impossible because of the range of practical competencies involved. So there are some fundamental barriers to the adoption of the whole spectrum of openness within nurses education. However, if we look in more detail at the sets of criteria we may also be able to see some possibilities.

Open access
A number of the criteria which emphasise the relevance of non-contiguity, such as the ability to study at the learner's own pace and place, clearly could be introduced to a number of nursing courses, and indeed form the basis for the second to first level conversion courses proposals made in 1989. Such proposals could fairly readily be extended to many other post-registration and pre-registration courses - it should be remembered that the Open University had a proposal for providing medical education. Similarly, the availability of a range of media for learning poses no fundamental problems.

Open pedagogy
A move to an open pedagogy would raise a number of more fundamental problems for nurse education which is based on the idea of acquiring a range of pre-set competencies. These competencies are prescribed by the statutory bodies in order to safeguard the public. However, certainly within post-registration courses and continuing education, there are moves towards a more learner centred approach which defines the practitioner as being best placed to define her learning needs and the competencies required in her situation. But there are examples which still represent a challenge to openness: for example, should a ward sister act as a mentor to her staff nurse who chooses to do a learning pack on primary nursing when the ward is struggling to introduce team nursing? Should she act as mentor to an enrolled nurse doing a learning pack on the administration of drugs when it is local policy that enrolled nurses do not administer drugs? What a nurse does in her own time in terms of personal development is a matter for her, but what she does in a work context is in time paid for by a health authority. The cession of control to registered nurses within continuing education would lead to a more diverse workforce and may raise issues of professional boundaries.

What could it achieve?

This is essentially a question which will be answered by practice, but the sum total of practical examples which have been analysed and documented is very small. Of course the papers in this book add dramatically to that total, but we are still in the realms of small scale experimental projects. However, we can suggest that there will be a two-fold answer which will be concerned first with the logistics of nurse education, and second with its aim.

Open learning has been presented as an answer to logistical problems in nurse education (Robinson 1988; Keane 1989). The advantages of open access within a scattered workforce with complex shift patterns is obvious. Similarly, many nurses are socially disadvantaged by their responsibilities at home and open learning provides access in this sense also. As the recruitment crisis deepens, the advantage to the employer of not having to release nurses from the workplace will become more pressing.

There has been less discussion of its potential in helping nurses acquire the competencies projected as essential for the nurse in the year 2000 However, research by Stainton Rogers (1986) shows that open learning is a very effective means of changing attitudes and this may be an essential part of the transformation of the nurse currently in practice. Moreover, it could be said that it is an effective method of bringing learning into the working situation where it can often most effectively take place, thus bridging the so-called theory-practice gap. A nurse can work directly on her competencies in the workplace using learning materials with a high interactive content; she can seize opportunities for learning - critical incidents - and explore her own performance in a reflective fashion. A workplace mentor can, through access to the learning materials, have an understanding of what and how the learner has been taught so that she can adapt her support appropriately.

Both the statutory bodies and the employers are promoting the idea of non-contiguous training for nurses. The statutory bodies through their approvals mechanisms have made it clear that they are happy to approve courses which are partly taught at a distance (and one such course is described in Chapter 12). The Health Pickup scheme is the vehicle for the employers to promote such training. The employers are unlikely to wish to adopt the broadest definitions of openness but it remains to be seen whether the statutory bodies will encourage the exploration of their full potential. The possibility that the statutory bodies and the NHSTA each promote open learning in order to deliver their particular message to the nurse efficiently and consistently is not an enticing one, as it involves the use of open learning for an essentially authoritarian purpose. However, if we consider the idea of open pedagogy, it is easy to recognise that this would suit the nurse of the future.

Notes

1. I am, of course, using pedagogy in the broadest sense here and encompassing all the attributes of andragogy.

References

Distance Learning Centre 1986 *Teaching Patients and Clients* Managing Care Pack 9, Distance Learning Centre, South Bank Polytechnic

Fricker J 1988 Open Learning: What's in it for Business? In Paine N (ed.) *Open Learning in Transition*. National Extension College

Hirst W 1986 Melbourne to Manchester: a look at openness in some open learning situations, *International Journal of Lifelong Education*, Vol 5 No 4 October - December pp327-46

Keane P 1989 Open learning: meeting educational needs, *Senior Nurse* 9, 2 pp12-14

Keegan D 1986 *The Foundations of Distance Education*, Croom Helm

Lentell H 1989 Open learning: breaking down the barriers, *Open Learning* 4, 1 pp58-9

Lewis R 1986 What is Open Learning? *Open Learning* 1, 2 pp12-17

Lewis R 1988 Open learning – the future. In Paine N (ed.) *Open Learning in Transition*.National Extension College

Lewis R and Spencer D 1986 *What is Open Learning?* Open Learning Guide 4, Council for Educational Technology

Marson S N undated *Teacher's Guide to Open/Distance Learning*. English National Board Learning Resources Unit

MSC 1988 *Ensuring Quality in Open Learning: A Handbook For Action* Manpower Services Commission.

Perry W 1976 *Open University*.The Open University Press

Robinson K M 1988 The distance learning mode diploma in nursing: a case study of collaboration. *International Journal of Nursing Studies* 25, 4 pp271-7

Rumble G 1989 'Open learning', 'distance learning', and the misuse of language, *Open Learning* 4, 2 pp28-36

Sewart D 1988 How student centred is the Open University? In Paine N (ed.) *Open Learning in Transition* National Extension College

Stainton Rogers W 1986 Changing attitudes through distance learning, *Open Learning,* 1, 3 pp12-17

Tait A 1988 Democracy in distance education and the role of tutorial and counselling services, *Journal of Distance Education 3 (1)*

Thorpe M Grugeon D (eds) 1987 *Open Learning for Adults*. Longman

Part 2:
The agony of production

3 Producing materials: an overview

Kate Robinson

Only a very small proportion of the people interested in open learning will ever need to master the technicalities of producing materials, and for them, there are a variety of other texts giving detailed advice (*see,* for example, Baath 1982; OU 1985; Lewis and Paine 1985; Rowntree 1986). A larger number of people may be involved peripherally in the planning or testing of materials and therefore need a broad knowledge of the whole process to understand where they 'fit in'. However, this chapter, and the following ones in this section, are mainly designed for the majority of consumers of open learning who will never be involved in production but who need to get a 'flavour' of the complexities of the production purpose for two reasons. First, so that they can make an informed decision about the quality of the materials being offered to them, and second, because an understanding of the complexities may persuade them *not* to embark on the process of production without a great deal of prior preparation and training.

The process of producing learning materials can be split into two parts – course creation and course production (*see,* for example Perry 1976; Perry and Rumble 1987). In broad terms, course creation is the label for the academic work involved in producing learning materials, whereas course production is the label for the reproduction of those materials. Another way of expressing the distinction is to say that course creation involves the making of one complete copy, at which point the course producers take over the reproduction of this 'master' copy. However, the two aspects are in practice usually intertwined and it is probably more useful to emphasise the importance of dialogue between course creators and producers, and the consequences which decisions about format, medium, style, etc. have for both the creators and the producers. So here I will use the generic term *production* for both phases and ask first: what and who are involved?

First, as in any educational programme, decisions have to be made about *what* you want to achieve, and second, *how* you are going to achieve it. Discussions over curriculum in any conventional course planning team will cover the same ground as in an open learning course team, but the aspect of '*how* you are going to achieve it' may be relatively neglected. For example, if a seminar method is proposed it is unlikely that the teacher will be asked to specify *exactly* how she proposes to conduct each seminar. The result is that many course submissions expound on the philosophy of the course and the syllabus but leave the actual 'how' issue buried in phrases like 'teaching will involve a mixture of tutorial, lecture and seminar work'. But in planning materials production, such decisions must be spelt out to a much greater degree of detail, partly because materials are usually created as a joint enterprise involving several people with different skills and each piece of the 'jigsaw' has to fit together, but also because they may have enormous financial implications.

Because a complex team of specialists is involved it will be useful to consider who they are. The teaching role remains, and is central to the team, but it is a much bigger team than in conventional teaching. The principal roles, depending on the choice of media, are:

- author
- editor/transformer
- graphic designer
- artist
- media consultant
- administrator

What, briefly, do these roles involve?

The roles in production

The *editor* is almost certainly the most important and the one whose expertise I would most want to have 'in-house'. She will certainly be an expert in copy-editing, that is checking a finished text for typographical and stylistic accuracy. But much more important than that, she will understand how to transform ideas into teaching materials – how to take a bald fact and turn it into a question; to insert an activity just when the learner is getting bored; to put in a self-check question just when the learner is getting confused. Very few authors have the experience and understanding of open learning to do that, and fewer still can do it to their own work. Classroom teachers are rarely challenged on the point of their favourite joke or the use of their favourite anecdote, but the editor will challenge each one, asking 'What do you really mean? What are you trying to achieve? What are the learners supposed to do?' A salutary exercise for any teacher! The role of the editor is explored further in Chapter 7.

The *graphic designer* will design the 'product' and is working on the side of the learner to make the package more intelligible and comprehensible. Ever since Marshall McLuhan told us that the medium was the message we have recognised the importance of presentation, but the graphic designer will persuade you that there are issues beyond 'Shall I write or type my OHPs?' She will advise on the use of fonts, of white space, of colour, of design, of the hundred and one things that turn ideas into packages. She will remind you that the audio-tape needs a label, that the package needs a wrapping, that the letter to your students should be in a complementary font to the text of the workbook. These should not be thought of as minor matters, as they are essential to the comfort, and therefore the motivation, of the learners and indeed to the whole educational experience. A change of font, for example, may signal to the learner a change in intellectual emphasis.

The *artist* has a smaller role than the graphic designer. She will be involved generally with producing illustrations for text including cartoons and line drawings. Some contact with the author remains essential because in producing a drawing from the author's note or 'stick' drawing the meaning may be changed. This is art in the service of education and it should be controlled by the author, although any sensible author will seek the artist's opinion on how a message can best be displayed.

The part played by the *media consultant* will depend on the media chosen; she will have expertise, usually, in media other than text, such as audio and video-tape. Except for people with a particular interest in such media, authors are dependent on the media consultant for good advice and would be wise to take it. Unfortunately, the advice is usually that the ideas and the budget are inherently incompatible. However, a good media consultant can often suggest an appropriate alternative which will achieve something worthwhile within budget. These issues are discussed further in Chapter 8.

The *administrator* is another very important person in production. Because so many people are involved and so many different activities need to be coordinated, good administration is essential. Let me give you just one example. For a simple text based package there might be, say, three authors, an editor and a graphic designer. All their meetings will have to be minuted and decisions recorded. Each author will write at least three drafts of their material, each of which will have to be recorded, duplicated and distributed for comment in-house. In addition, distribution of some drafts will involve external critical readers and learner groups – all of whom have to be briefed and coordinated. All comments likewise have to be recorded, duplicated and distributed. Once a draft has been finalised, permissions have to be sought for copyright, artists have to be employed, artwork has to be recorded, duplicated and distributed. The administrator is therefore the backbone of the course production team and this is reflected in the fact that the Open University has created a new grade of staff to fulfil many of these functions – the course manager. In small organisations the administrator will also liaise with the people involved in the reproduction of the master copy, such as printers. However, larger organisations will usually have a project control department which overviews and schedules the whole process.

The course team

How do all these people work together? The Open University model, which has been widely adopted, is to have a course team which works together throughout the production of the course and deals with all aspects of production.

> Essentially each team was to consist of three groups of staff: academics, educational technologists and BBC production staff... the course team must not only create a course of quality and standard, they must create it at a time and a price consistent with the efficient functioning of the University as a whole.
>
> Perry 1976

The exact way in which teams function varies even within the Open University. Some teams work so closely that the eventual text is credited simply to the course team. Other teams effectively delegate the writing task, within defined limits, to one member who retains the individual authorship – the normal form of words is something like 'prepared for the Course Team by Amy Bloggins'.

However, the Open University course team model is not the only possible way of organising the necessary human resources. Other models use much smaller course teams or use external authors and consultants working with a very small internal core team. Figure 3.1 sets out some of the possible models but these are, of course ideal types and in practice there are many more permutations.

The advantage of using external authors and consultants is that different specialists can be recruited as required. For the production of the Open University course P553, *A Systematic Approach to Nursing Care*, for example, apart from the internal academic who chaired the course team, all the academic members were recruited from outside the Open University. The Distance Learning Centre (DLC) also uses an extensive network of external authors but they are not generally involved in the internal course team but simply submit work according to a specification. The disadvantage of using external

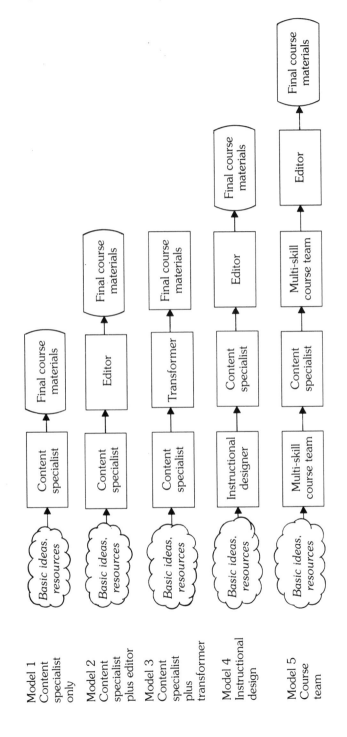

Figure 3.1 Course team models

authors is that writing open learning materials is so specialised an activity that external authors rarely have the appropriate skills, and much editing and 'transforming' of materials needs to be done subsequently. This may lengthen the production time scale and consequently reduce some of the savings made by using consultants rather than maintaining a full-time academic team.

The course specification

What are the issues which the course team has to address? Whatever their chosen style of working, they have to agree a course specification. However, before they can make those decisions, they need detailed information on the resources available. Necessary resources include a substantial budget for staff costs and printing costs, but another less obvious consideration is the human expertise at your disposal. Expertise in open learning in *general* is readily available, but not in open learning for *nursing*. The lack of such skilled personnel is likely to inhibit the development of any project, as expertise will have to be 'home grown'.

The detail involved in the course specification should include the following as a minimum:

- The aims of the material: these can be formulated as objectives but there is considerable controversy within open learning about how far the use of objectives is appropriate. Certainly it is important to consider how far a *general* set of objectives is compatible with ideas about promoting *individual* growth and personal development.
- The intended study time: it is difficult to be accurate (and it is not always necessary to be so) but you do need to know whether the materials should take two hours or two weeks to study.
- A profile of the targeted learner, including ability level, previous experience, and motivation.
- Whether any human support will be available to the learner, such as a teacher or workplace mentor.
- The type of media to be used: choosing usually from a basic menu of text, audio-tape, video-tape, interactive video and computer programs. However, even the bald statement 'text' must be further refined to describe the length, the style of writing, the number and type of illustrations, etc.
- A pedagogic specification showing how the learner will relate to the materials and how flexible the materials may be.
- An outline design specification, giving some idea of whether photographs, line drawings, etc can be used.
- The production timetable. Statistically, a group of apes could

write an excellent open learning text given sufficient millennia, but normally the timetable is a great deal shorter and decisions therefore need to be made about who is available for authoring, how the job will be allocated, etc.

• The quality control system: this is likely to involve the testing of the material by 'subject' experts and by representative users.

I now look at some of these aspects in more detail.

The targeted learner

Because of the costs of producing effective learning materials, they are designed for use by large numbers of students and it is therefore difficult to define your 'targeted' learner very precisely. This problem is exacerbated because of the emphasis on open access. Many conventional courses 'weed out' students who they don't think are quite right for the course, either by a simple rejection or by fairly directive 'counselling out'. But if an open learning system is designed to give everyone a chance, then the materials should be accessible in an intellectual as well as a physical sense to all the learners.

However, it could be argued, as with any vocational course, that the learner is not the only consumer of your learning material and the needs of their employers also need to be taken into account. This aspect may be exaggerated in the case of open learning materials because *first,* the high cost of production means that there may be a consortium of sponsors, not all of whom will agree about the desired end product and *second,* the learning materials will be highly visible. It is this visibility which sometimes subjects producers of open learning materials to unreasonable criticism and thereby renders them cautious. The Open University in particular has received criticism about its published materials and is consequently extremely careful. This problem has been described by Perry (1976) as occurring very early on in the life of the Open University, although he notes that they had, at the time of writing, avoided a major confrontation with the government, firms or public organisations. Politics (with a big 'P') is perhaps less likely to be an issue in nursing education but there is an issue of how far materials should represent the views of any particular group or faction. To take one example, should materials assume that professionalisation is to be welcomed: should they use the word 'profession' or the rather less loaded 'occupation'? Such semantic issues are relatively unimportant when any individual teacher might only reach an audience of say twenty or thirty or a hundred learners in a year, and that within one district. But when materials such as *A Systematic Approach to Nursing Care* have an estimated readership of over 60,000 over four years, then there may be conflict over the control of the content.

The type of media

Text is the obvious choice but it is not the only choice, so what are the criteria to be used? Learner needs should be the most important criterion, answering the question: how would it be most helpful for the learner to have this presented? This can be particularly important with aspects of the course which are most closely involved in 'real-life' situations. A discussion of the nursing process, for instance, should utilise documentation which reflects what is occurring on the wards. P553, *A Systematic Approach to Nursing Care* incorporates a set of 'case files' which includes patient details and notes in a realistic format.

However, the choice of media cannot be made in isolation from some concern about how the student is likely to cope with it. Video is certainly not universally available and neither are computers – certainly not ones able to use appropriate software. In addition, the *time* of use is important. Learners may want to study at home rather than in a library where audio-visual equipment might be available. Study in a nursing situation is perfectly possible using text, but might be more conspicuous or complicated with other technology.

Another important, and sometimes pre-eminent, criterion is cost. Some media are a great deal more expensive to use than others. Anything involving video is still very expensive, although the costs are reducing. However, audio-tape can be fairly cheap and cheerful and provide some variety in a text based course. The DLC Diploma in Nursing, for example, uses an audio-tape of interviews with various people – including a group of schoolchildren – to run alongside a text based module on *Images of Nursing* (Robinson and Vaughan 1988). The problems of choosing appropriate media will be pursued in Chapter 8.

Pedagogic specification

This is the aspect of course production which will reflect the pedagogic views of the course team and determine where your materials will come within the family of 'open learning'. Materials can simply impart information and use in-text activities or self-assessment questions to help the learner work through the information. Alternatively they can entice the learner into a journey of self-discovery and skill acquisition in partnership with the author which will involve participation in more complex activities and more detailed contributions by the learner. The issue of whether the materials will be linear or non-linear, the style of presentation (chatty, academic, didactic, etc.) must be decided, and if there is more than one author, the degree of consistency which is required is also important.

The issue of the required homogeneity of style is an interesting one which concerns consumers as well as producers of materials. Thorpe comments about text writing in the Open University:

> I think there has been a change in this respect among Open University course teams at least, which reflects the accumulation of years of experience with a very wide range of subject areas and course designs. It is probably true to say in the early years it was thought important that all units should achieve as near as possible a 'house style' of impersonal clarity and rationality, and that the course materials as a whole should have a uniform style. There is now a more sophisticated grasp of the difficulties of writing good teaching material, and of the indissolubility of style and content. Perhaps more important has been the realisation that for many students, differences of style can be stimulating and that units which give a sense of the personality behind the writing can make as positive a contribution to learning as others which do not.

Thorpe 1988

The production timetable

The production of open learning materials is basically an industrial process, despite the educational context. And for it to be efficient, each aspect of the work has to be very tightly scheduled. Slippage in any part of the system is potentially catastrophic and costly.

It might be thought that authoring will go to schedule if experienced teachers are used. After all, teachers are very used to being timetabled and begin to take it for granted. If they are scheduled to teach 'Research methods' at three o'clock on Wednesday afternoon then, in general, that's when it will happen regardless of whether fifteen hours or fifteen minutes has gone into the preparation for it. Most teachers are reasonably expert at 'muddling' through and if things don't go terribly well in one session then they can often be repaired later. However, an open learning context presents different problems. First, there is the pressure of the unseen audience of hundreds and thousands which, in theory are a spur to optimising standards but in practice may lead to complete 'writer's block'. If the author is in a situation where she is trying to combine open learning authoring with teaching face-to-face and dealing with the normal run of learners problems, then she will find it enormously difficult to switch from reacting to the learners making current demands to proactive work for learners in the future whom she may never meet.

It is difficult to generalise about production time scales, except to say that they are almost always longer than anticipated, and of course it depends on which events are included in the timing and which methods are used in production. But in my experience it is difficult to go through all the stages of the basic text production process in less than one year, and two to three years is a much more realistic schedule for anything of any size. The steps of the production process for text based material are outlined in the next section.

Production stages

The following specification of production stages comes from the DLC. Other production centres will use slightly different stages but the principles will be similar. The system of drafts was developed by the Open University and has been widely adopted elsewhere.

1 Basic specification produced, including aims and objectives.
2 Author identified; objectives and content negotiated; author briefed about style; written directions given.
3 Draft 0 produced, ie a statement of intent or outline. Discussed by course team.
4 Draft 1 produced, ie the first presentation of 'complete' material. Discussed by course team and changes negotiated with author.
5 Draft 2 produced incorporating the suggested changes and sent for developmental testing, critical reading and external appraisal.
6 Comments collated and reviewed, author briefed.
7 Draft 3 produced, reviewed by course team and either accepted or further revision proposed.
8 Final vetting by external appraiser; handover to editor.
9 Editor liaises with graphic designer and printing team (who should also have been involved in planning at earlier stages).
10 Handover to printer and the cycle of proof correction.
11 Publication.

Quality control

Systematic quality control in conventional teaching is really only in its infancy. In nurse education, for example, the English National Board began to look at performance indicators in the late 1980s. However, most producers of open learning materials have paid great attention to this aspect. Much of the credit for this must go to the Open University which has from the first insisted on excellence. There are two aspects to quality control of content in the production stage:

- critical reading by experts
- study by 'typical' learners.

Exactly how the first aspect is managed will depend on how the course team is constituted; critical reading by experts should start in-house with the sharing of drafts amongst colleagues for comment and rewriting, but it should always be followed by the perusal of drafts by experts from outside the institution. They can be asked both to check the contents of the material for accuracy and bias but also to evaluate it as teaching material. This latter aspect may prove difficult; critical readers may find it impossible to think like a learner and may comment 'this is too simple' or 'why didn't you pursue this idea further' without really thinking through what can reasonably be expected of a learner in the time available. The 'high profile' aspect of learning materials also comes to the fore again. Critical readers may have a slight worry that these materials may be seen by people who might 'judge' the state of nursing knowledge by them; they think that they should reflect the 'best' in nursing. But materials have to connect with the learners and *their* concerns otherwise they may leave them far behind. Most critical readers are asked to look at just one particular aspect of the materials where they have expertise. However, there is often also an appraiser, who oversees the whole rather than just the parts to make sure that it 'hangs together' both in terms of a correct approach to the topic and of being appropriate teaching material for the intended audience.

Developmental testing by learners is equally important, especially in the early stages of an open learning production programme when the authors might not have got a 'feel' for their audience. The learners should ideally reflect all the possible types who might eventually do the course and therefore, for most courses in nursing, just one group of testers is insufficient. The DLC's Managing Care programme was very extensively tested throughout the country and the feedback led to some radical redrafting. However, getting sufficiently critical feedback can be a problem – nurses seem conditioned to be polite. Ideally, of course, the author should go and meet the developmental testers to extract more acerbic comments but this isn't always possible. However, it is very salutary for any author to listen to learners discussing a draft – what seemed obvious to the author may be highly obscure to the learner. A more sophisticated type of developmental testing involves learners working through an entire course, that is the materials plus what support would normally be available, in a simulation of the real thing. Thorpe (1988) describes such a model of testing used within the Open University to overcome the problems of less structured testing, which she formulates as:

- the testers are not comparable with eventual learners
- the testers do not use the materials and try to learn 'for real'
- a high proportion of testers drops out
- the feedback is inconsistent
- the data will relate only to the learners' views on the materials and *not* whether they have learnt anything.

Despite the inadequacies of some models of developmental testing it is an extremely important part of the quality assurance process. However, it is responsible for a major part of the cost of production, both because there are direct costs (travel costs, duplication of materials, etc.) and indirect, but substantial, costs of lengthened timescales.

Making or borrowing?

The Open University has put a great deal of effort into developing ideas about the production of materials and clearly has a great deal of expertise. It is regularly criticised, however, for being too expensive, for 'making a fuss about nothing'. 'Anyone', it is said, 'can produce learning materials, especially in these days of desk-top publishing'. Certainly the introduction of sophisticated document processing software at a reasonable price has opened up a number of possibilities, and many nurse teachers are producing learning materials for their students using the technology available in their school or college. Sometimes, they are keen to recover their costs by selling these materials elsewhere. However, as soon as the materials are used in a context not controlled directly by the author then they become stand-alone products which, if their users are not to be confused, mis-informed and generally 'put-off' open learning, must meet the sort of production standards described above, which are expensive. The Open Tech programme, for example, started with great ideas about how the costs of production could be reduced, but many projects learnt the hard way that quality also suffered, although simple training materials are cheaper to produce than materials dealing with complex ideas and competencies.

Because of the complex nature of production and the high set-up cost of establishing an in-house production unit, the obvious solution within nurse education (cf Dixon 1987) is to buy-in materials from specialist production centres such as the Open University and the Distance Learning Centre. These materials need not be produced specifically for nursing; they could be interdisciplinary or concerned with a generic issue such as management. There are a number of data bases which give information about materials which are available (for example, MARIS-NET), including a specialist nursing facility run by the ENB Resource and Careers Service. However, all such materials should be evaluated with regard to the nature of the production process and particularly the quality control process. Information about this may not be given explicitly but acknowledgements may be made to teams of developmental testers and to critical readers. Unfortunately it is not always easy to know how well materials will function in practice just by looking at them, but producers should be willing to pass on the names of other users who may have helpful advice. It would be extremely useful if producers produced more accounts of how the materials have been used and in what contexts.

Materials imported into a particular situation might need to be adapted for use in a number of ways. Again, there is a useful literature on the process of adaptation (Lewis and Paine 1986; Stainton Rogers 1987). As Stainton Rogers notes, some teachers feel almost compelled to change materials before they can use them, either to prove their autonomy or their conscientiousness but there are also sound educational reasons for making different degrees of change. She categorises these changes as:

1 *Transformation*, which consists of re-working and re-formulation such as rewriting text, using a different medium, changing the form (eg putting a diagram onto an OHP transparency). Changes may include level of difficulty, degree of specificity, or the context used.
2 *Selection*, where some parts of the material are chosen as appropriate, and others discarded, to ensure that students only tackle that which is appropriate.
3 *Augmentation* by introducing additional material or input, to make the materials more up-to-date, topical, locally relevant, or to increase conceptual depth or specificity.
4 *Integration* whereby materials are linked to other teaching inputs so that students experience coherent learning rather than a series of isolated and even conflicting elements.

Stainton Rogers 1987

She argues that the first two categories are simply possibilities which may be considered and need to be handled with care: however, the last two categories should always be carried out when materials are brought into a situation for which they were not specifically designed. However, this takes us into the realms of learner support which are dealt with in Part Three.

The chapters which follow in this part look in more detail at some of the issues of production and will be useful both to those who want to become producers and those who need to be informed consumers. However, it is important to emphasise that, although good materials will enter into dialogue with the learner, materials on their own do not constitute an open learning system; the second, and equally important part of the system, is the support which is available to the learner, and that is discussed in Part Three.

References

Baath J A 1982 Some possibilities of attempting to fulfil instructional functions. In Holmberg B and Baath J A *Distance Education: a short handbook*. Liber-harmods, Malmo

Dixon K 1987 *Implementing Open Learning in Local Authority Institutions*. Further Education Unit/Open Learning Branch (MSC)

Lewis R and Paine N 1985 *How to Communicate with the Learner*. Council for Educational Technology, Open Learning Guide 6

Lewis R and Paine N 1986 *How to Find and Adapt Materials and Elect Media*. Open Learning Guide 8. Council for Educational Technology

OU 1984 P553 *A Systematic Approach to Nursing Care*. The Open University Press

OU 1985 P517 *Making Self-instructional Materials for Adults, Checklist 3*. The Open University Press

Perry W 1976 *Open University*. The Open University Press

Perry W and Rumble G 1987 *A Short Guide to Distance Education*. International Extension College. 2nd edition

Robinson K S M and Vaughan B 1988 *Images of Nursing*. Distance Learning Centre

Rowntree D 1986 *Teaching Through Self-Instruction*. Kogan Page

Stainton Rogers W 1987 Adapting materials for alternative use. In Thorpe M and Grugeon D (eds.) *Open Learning for Adults*. Longman

Thorpe M 1988 *Evaluating Open and Distance Learning*. Longman

MARIS-NET
Run by MARIS (Materials and Resources Information Service) 1 St Mary's Street, Ely CB4 4ER

4 Setting up a production unit: issues and challenges

Elisabeth Clark and Kate Robinson

The Distance Learning Centre (DLC), at South Bank Polytechnic, was one of over 140 projects originally funded by the Manpower Services Commission (MSC) through its Open Tech initiative. The project began in April 1984 and was funded, on a pump-priming basis, for three years only. If it was to survive, it had to become self-sustaining either through sales and fee income or by attracting alternative sources of subsidy. Since the account of the first years of the project, which forms the core of this chapter, has been jointly written by the first two directors of the centre, it will inevitably be a partial (in both senses of the word) account. Nevertheless, we have tried to use the account as a vehicle for a discussion of a number of issues which are relevant to any producer of open learning materials on whatever scale.

The original brief for the project was to develop materials for the Diploma in Nursing (University of London) but it was by no means clear what form these would take or how they would be distributed. In short, there was no realistic specification to follow when the first director, who had not been involved in the negotiations for the contract, came into post. While this could be construed as a disadvantage – and at the time it seemed pretty catastrophic – it actually gave the room for manoeuvre that was essential for success. A very important early decision taken by the DLC was that the project should aim to become an independent self-sustaining unit after the expiration of the contract. This was not the simple decision which it sounds, as many people involved in the Open Tech saw the project as a means of getting a specific set of materials developed to support existing teaching and had no desire to create a permanent unit. The decision was prompted in part by professional considerations: it seemed important that there should be a specialist producer of open learning materials for nursing (the Open University, at that time, was reluctant to take on that role). However, it must also be said that the decision was prompted in part by staff considerations. All the staff for the DLC were appointed from outside the host institution and their jobs depended on its survival. This doubtless encouraged a desire to create a permanent unit. So, the essential problem was how to become self-sustaining within three years *while* remaining within the parameters of the Open Tech contract (which could be cancelled pretty well at any time) – *and* within the policies and structures of the Polytechnic, which were not geared to open learning (indeed there was a degree of frank antagonism to open learning within the Polytechnic). Decisions had to be made quickly as the contract had begun in March 1984 but it had taken until the very end of July of that year to get a Director in post, and large sums of money could not be vired between years.

Aims of the DLC

The policies adopted by the DLC at the start formed the basis of all future work. To begin, it was decided that the DLC would both create learning materials and provide support to the learner. Hence, academic staff would have direct responsibilities for supporting individual learners as well as for authoring materials. The model for this was, of course, the Open University, from whence the first Director had come, rather than the philosophy of the Open Tech, which envisaged a separation between producers and distributors of open learning materials. The Diploma materials which the DLC would produce would form the basis of an open learning mode of presentation for the Diploma, run by the DLC.

As with any other institution planning to run the Diploma, we had to begin extensive discussions with the University of London in order to obtain validation. The outcome of these discussions could not be prejudged and therefore the whole timetable of the project was in jeopardy. Furthermore, the University of London had little or no prior experience of open learning and therefore subjected the DLC's proposals to a thorough and rigorous validation. Whilst the University was very sympathetic, in their view the validation of an open learning course had to include appraisal of the materials. For obvious logistical and financial reasons, the DLC was unwilling and unable to produce specific materials prior to validation. This is an important issue in the validation of open learning courses, since the DLC took the view that it was being asked effectively to teach the course prior to obtaining validation and that this was unreasonable in comparison with the standards required of any other institution seeking validation for a conventional version of the Diploma. The situation was exacerbated by the fact that the agreed funding from MSC was most generous in the first year, but decreased each year on the assumption that income generation could fill the gap. But we could not rely on fee income in 1987 for a course which might not receive validation by then – or indeed ever, so we needed a safety net.

The safety net was to be a development programme for nurses based on a number of short packs or modules of learning materials which would be available on a 'pick and mix' basis. This kind of 'menu' of opportunities unfettered by the course rules and regulations of an external validating body was in accord with the philosophy of the Open Tech and they were happy to renegotiate the contract on that basis. The new plan envisaged production for this programme, which would not require conventional academic validation, displacing some of the production for the Diploma which it would subsequently subsidise through sales income. It was hoped that some of the short modules might even be incorporated into the Diploma programme. A similar dual use of material was developed for Unit 5 of the Diploma – the research element. A suggestion from staff of Essex Institute of Higher Education that there was a market for a set of open learning materials on research led to Unit 5 being developed as the 'Research Awareness Programme' and made available for independent sale.

So the original plan for producing materials for the Diploma had been transformed into a long term plan involving at least three separate programmes:

- the Diploma in Nursing (University of London) to be taught by the DLC;
- the Managing Care programme of short modules to be available on a 'pick and mix' basis, with the possibility that study of a series of modules could lead to some form of certification at a later date;
- the Research Awareness Programme of separate modules, again available on a 'pick and mix' basis, but together forming a complete syllabus on the use of research in nursing.

As well as the specific focus on course production, we also saw that we would have to spend a lot of time educating the potential market about open learning. This was partly for obvious business reasons – you can't sell to people who don't understand your product – but also because we saw one of the roles of a specialist open learning centre being to enter into a dialogue with the target occupation to discuss the potential and limitations of the methodology of open learning.

In summary, these early planning stages gave rise to a series of implicit aims, which were later explicitly stated as follows:

- the production and distribution of open learning materials
- the presentation of open and distance learning courses
- research into open learning in vocational training in the

health care sector
- raising awareness of the potential of open learning amongst all categories of staff in the health care sector.

Robinson 1986

The last of these aims committed the staff of the Centre to a substantial programme of workshops, open days and other public relations activities. Although there is some return in terms of subsequent orders, the commitment has always been to that of promoting open learning in general, rather than DLC products and services in particular, and this work has always placed a great strain on the Centre.

Solving problems by increasing commitments, rather than by lessening them, might seem a strange way to proceed but it seemed at the time – and we find no reason to doubt it since – that open learning depends on economies of scale. A small open learning production centre is almost a contradiction in terms. Long-term survival depended on finding a cost effective size, although we would not claim that this has yet been achieved.

Staffing

Having decided what we were going to do, the next problem was to appoint a team to do it. The original contract called for a substantial team of staff but this would impose an enormous drain on resources in the long term. All staff, including the Director, were appointed on short term contracts, renewable each year, and it would therefore have been possible to recruit staff for only short periods of time, but this seemed neither acceptable nor practical. It was not acceptable to ask staff to commit themselves to the project with a view to getting rid of them when income diminished (unless, perhaps, they were seconded by their current employers). Practically, it took staff a long time to gain expertise in distance learning and this expertise had to be retained. Consequently, a small team was recruited, which we aimed to retain and keep intact.

But who was the team to consist of? What staff are necessary to run an open learning production unit? Again, there was little help to be found in the original contract as it omitted important roles such as editors and administrators. These proved to be key appointments for the success or otherwise of the project. The administrator is essential for the production side, for day to day contact with consumers and for keeping financial records – tasks usually done by distinct teams of staff but in a small team subsumed within one job description. In theory some of these jobs, such as financial administration, could have been done by departments within the Polytechnic, but in practice they were not geared to giving the sort of accurate and detailed information that was necessary. A small open learning production centre which is organised as a distinct cost-centre must operate as a small business. However, unlike a small business, we were often constrained by the practices and policies of the larger institution. For example, we were required, by the Polytechnic, to follow a complex appointment procedure, the costs of which the Centre was required to bear. We found it difficult to operate within the standard Polytechnic role descriptions and related salaries, which bore little or no resemblance to the work we were doing.

While larger organisations (such as the Open University) are able to fund a relatively large number of permanent staff, smaller scale operations typically find the funding of such posts to be a considerable drain on resources and are unlikely to be able to support many permanent appointments. Even by 1988, four years after the start of the project, only one third of the DLC core staff team had moved to permanent contracts.

Even after entering this phase of the development of the Centre, with the appointment of a small core of permanent staff, the need to recruit individuals on short-term contracts remains. Specifically, there is a need to appoint people to work full-time on individual projects as the funds for these become available. At the DLC, each programme area has a full-time project-leader/course director who assumes responsibility for curriculum development, structuring course content, commissioning external authors, developing course materials and for the day to day administration of the programme. Ideally, such people will have recent experience in teaching and curriculum design but may have little or no background in open learning. They are thus likely to rely heavily on guidance and support from the permanent in-house experts and it is, therefore, necessary to recognise the time and resource implications of this mode of operation. The major benefit of such fixed-term posts to the project is the flexibility they afford, enabling specific expertise to be bought in as and when it is needed (assuming, of course, that it is available).

A scarcity of full-time staff means that it is not possible to write and edit all the materials in-house and any small scale unit has, therefore, to rely heavily on the use of external contributors. A nucleus of internal staff must work alongside and co-ordinate the activities of a much larger number of external authors and editors. Certainly the short-term appointment of specialists who are commissioned to produce a given piece of work offers even greater flexibility. In this way, we utilised the intellectual resources of other institutions. In fact, some individuals employed as external consultants would not, for a variety of reasons, have been available to teach the material on a face-to-face basis on a conventional course. Either their work commitments precluded it or they lived a long way from the DLC – even overseas – but were able, with careful briefing and support to prepare materials. As Robinson (1988) remarks 'It is often not fully appreciated that the flexibility inherent in distance learning which is such an advantage to the students is also of great benefit to the staff.'

However, the reliance on external authors can also give rise to a number of problems as well as an issue of morality. In terms of morality, using staff in this way is essentially parasitic. The recruiting organisation does not pay for staff development, for personal growth, for the experience necessary to produce the expertise, rather it pays merely for the time taken for this particular task. In the business world this essential element may be costed in, but fees paid for educational work are rarely sufficient.

The *first* of the more practical problems is that external authors often take much longer (than experienced internal authors) to prepare materials, which may in addition require extensive rewriting. *Second,* the experts in any field tend to be heavily committed and may therefore, even with the best of intentions, be unable to devote sufficient time to meet critical production schedules. In our experience, no amount of cajoling, nor the use of penalty clauses in contracts, are effective in solving this problem. Furthermore, undue pressure on individuals can result in them pulling out altogether. The only partial remedy is to ensure that the writing brief is extremely detailed, which at least cuts out unnecessary effort and often seems less daunting to an inexperienced author. *Third,* even outstanding academics with an excellent reputation in their field, and a long list of publications to their name, can find it difficult to communicate their knowledge and expertise and create successful interactive learning materials. The fact is that this requires skills very different from those associated with either formal lecturing or academic writing – probably something more akin to journalism with an emphasis on communication. The text needs to be highly interactive, encouraging students to think through specific issues for themselves and relate them to their own situation The style needs to be friendly, rather than pedantic, whilst not being patronising. It is also important to structure material carefully and signpost intentions (see Chapter 7)

There are a number of excellent texts available which help authors to develop an appropriate style (Rowntree 1986; Lewis and Paine 1986). However, in our experience, even with the aid of such guides and very careful briefing and support, some authors are clearly surprised by the challenges presented. They frequently find that it requires them to rethink their subject and how it should be presented at a fairly fundamental level. Writing interactive materials also has the salutary effect of showing up the limitations of much conventional face-to-face teaching. It is clear that many external authors find it either extremely difficult or, at best, very time consuming to produce such materials. Indeed Rowntree (1986) has estimated that every hour of study time may take between 50-100 (or more) hours of time to develop and produce. A modest fee negotiated for, say, five hours of study time can begin to look decidedly inadequate. It is likely that many authors would never have agreed to become involved in the first place if they had been aware of the time required. In addition to this, many authors find it hard to come to terms with constructive criticism made by critical readers and developmental testers. Authors may be reluctant to modify their work or allow others to do so, since this may be deemed to interfere with their academic freedom.

Course teams

While some of these difficulties may reflect the fact that open learning is a relative newcomer to nursing, and the pool of skills should expand in the future, the problem is unlikely to be resolved in the short term. Given these difficulties, heavy reliance has to be placed on what Rowntree (1986) calls 'transformers', that is, people who are skilled communicators who liaise with subject specialists, helping them to express the key concepts and ideas in ways that can be easily understood. Without 'transformer' skills (and even with them) a project is likely to end up with filing cabinets full of materials which cannot be used without a considerable amount of reworking and, thus, a commitment of further resources. Even in an ideal situation, it is worth stressing that a high proportion of draft material is – and should be – thrown away.

At the DLC we have experimented with a number of different models. Initially we adopted the course team model, as pioneered by the Open University. A course team typically consisted of one or more course authors, people with production experience, an editor, a designer and an administrator. The team meet regularly to plan and oversee the development of course materials within a specific programme area. Materials would be discussed by the group as a whole and detailed suggestions made for amendment. Certainly the Open University experience suggests that course teams can operate efficiently and constructively to facilitate the development and production of high quality course materials.

Initially, each of the three major programmes at the DLC established their own course team, but it soon became obvious that such methods could not be sustained within a small project. There were simply insufficient full-time members of staff available to operate a full course team for each programme. Key individuals were spending nearly all their time attending course team meetings, leaving little or no time for the rest of their work. Moreover, it proved impossible to use external consultants on course teams because the pressure of their other commitments made it impossible to timetable meetings. One strategy developed to deal with this problem is the writing cluster: pairs or small groups of authors, including wherever possible the programme director, work closely together supporting each other whilst also liaising with at least one other member of the production team. Another useful model is that of 'yoking' an external author with an experienced academic editor or internal academic staff member so that they can develop materials together. However, asking internal academics to devote much of their time to academic editing of other people's work is eventually destructive of creativity and enthusiasm – getting the balance right is important.

Quality control

Although the MSC has subsequently taken a great interest in issues of quality control, producing the handbook *Ensuring Quality in Open Learning* in 1988, this was not entirely apparent in 1984. At the time there was a general feeling that there was nothing much to this open learning business, and while the Open University may have got the quality right, they spent far too much money and time achieving that result. Ratios of production time to study time as low as 3:1 were being urged on project managers. However, the DLC from the start insisted on a complex and time consuming quality control mechanism, partly because of the Open University experience of the Director, but also because it was felt that the success of open learning in nursing depended on the obvious quality of these materials. A failure here would be likely to set the 'cause' back many years. The Open University had set a quality standard and the DLC had to meet or better it – but with far fewer resources!

Quality control for open learning rests on three systems – one internal and two external. Internally there needs to be considerable discussion and debate about the materials; ideas must be knocked about, tested in debate and found wanting. Materials should go through several draft stages – a minimum of three – before publication. The discussion above shows that the internal procedures were to some extent jeopardised by resource constraints, so the external systems became more important. External assessment consists of developmental testing and critical reading. Developmental testing involves groups of 'typical' learners working through the materials, usually at the stage of the second draft. For critical reading, subject experts and educationalists are asked to comment on the draft materials, usually at the stages of the second and third drafts.

It was difficult in the early period of the project to show developmental testers and critical readers what the final product would look like – indeed we often didn't know ourselves. Sometimes the rather scruffy double-spaced typed manuscripts with little or no artwork left a great deal to the imagination. However, once the first finished example of materials from a particular programme was available then testers had a clearer indication of the high standards aimed for. It is important to involve members of the target audience as much as possible and as early as possible in the process of developing materials for two reasons. First, because they will help you to check whether the material is at the right level and appears credible, especially in occupational terms. Second, as Webberley (1988) comments, it offers you a means of introducing the learner's voice into the pack through using their comments and anecdotes.

Developmental testers have been used for all the material, although with less emphasis in the case of the Diploma. Because the Diploma material addresses an agreed syllabus the content cannot be freely changed in response to the students, and we became more familiar with the appropriate level and style as we wrote more Diploma material and began to meet the students and assess their work. For the Managing Care programme, however, developmental testing remains vital: each new module presents a new set of problems and concerns which can only be resolved by 'fieldwork'. And it is through such fieldwork that we realised what a heterogeneous occupation nursing is. The problems of addressing all the different specialties, areas of work, philosophies, traditions, etc. were, and are, almost insuperable, not least because each faction demands its own overt recognition within the material. To give just one very basic example, should we refer to patients or clients? A majority of the team came from a community background and favoured 'client', but the members with a hospital background felt that this would lack credibility for many nurses. The problem remained unresolved as can be seen by the title of one of the Managing Care modules: *Teaching Patients and Clients* (DLC 1986). These problems also colour the choice of critical readers who should ideally come from a variety of backgrounds. The biggest problem with expert advice is remembering that the countries which make up the United Kingdom differ considerably in the way their health system is organised and managed and in the legal system which controls it. Even the Open University has been caught out by problems with legal differences. Running a national open learning system requires a ruthless rejection of ethnocentrism.

Production

Open learning packs typically employ a wide range of teaching media including print, audio and video material and computer based learning (*see* Chapter 8). However, because we were working within a very restricted budget, we had to focus on 'low' technology media such as print and audio-tape. They have, of course, the great advantage of being accessible to most students, and it was this aspect which was emphasised by both the *Nursing Times* cover, which showed a learner and her workbook in the bath, and the *Nursing Standard* cover, which showed a Managing Care workbook being shared between a patient in bed and her nurses.

However, despite being relatively low cost, the financial implications of various formats need to be investigated very carefully, and this is where dialogue with the production specialists proved vital. The original plan was for the DLC to generate camera ready copy using in-house computer facilities which were shared with other projects. The specialist staff such as designers and word-processor operators were also to be shared. This plan ran into trouble straight away on a number of counts. First, and most important, the computer hardware and software then available could not produce sufficient quality of presentation for our needs. Second, the idea of sharing production staff assumed a surplus rather than a scarce commodity. None of the projects succeeded in forward scheduling with any degree of accuracy – the variables were just too great and we were too inexperienced – and all of them demanded that resources should be devoted to *their* project the instant they needed them. This was not simply a matter of childish tantrums but of economic necessity; we come again to the fact that these projects had to run as small businesses – they simply could not afford time delays.

Because of the problems of limited internal resources, and also because the camera ready copy was not offering the quality of reproduction or the flexibility of layout that was needed, we decided to rely on traditional printing methods although doing some of the layout work in-house to save money. This system worked reasonably well for a while, although there were always problems and the time scales involved often seemed excessive.

Certainly the negotiations with the printers were complex and, in our experience, best left to experts. But the academics had a great deal to learn about printing simply because you cannot make reasonable choices about layout, style, or even contents, in a vacuum; you have to think about what something will cost in a way that is unfamiliar to most teachers. To choose, for example, to put key words in the margin – a simple device to help students find their way around a text – would involve complex 'pasting-up' by the graphic artist and thus time and money. 'Was it worth it? Could the money be better spent on some other device?' – the discussions could be endless. One particularly notable set of discussions revolved around the colours for the front covers of the Managing Care workbooks. They were eventually chosen after days of debate to reflect the themes of contents (the only one we balked at was purple for death!) but we have yet to meet any consumer who has actually noticed them. Packaging is extremely important to both the purchaser and the user of the material but how many resources it should absorb is a very difficult question.

Each of the three programmes has a different format. The Managing Care study packs are beautifully presented with spiral binding, glossy covers, a lot of visual stimuli such as cartoons, photos and 'thought bubbles', and space left for learners to record their responses to specific activities. Each pack consists of at least two parts, a workbook and one other component such as a reader or an audio-tape. Overall, this method of production creates a general feeling of quality. The relatively high demand for these materials makes this method of production viable although the higher production costs must be reflected in the price. The Research Awareness materials, however, are more functional with a view to minimising production costs wherever possible. For example, feedback from developmental testing consistently commented on the desirability of having the offprints (a collection of published materials that are needed to complete certain of the activities) printed separately, which would enable the reader to consult the two simultaneously side-by-side. However, the cost implications of providing two separate components to each module did not allow us to do that; instead the offprints were printed on coloured paper and enclosed in the middle of the stapled module so that they could be pulled out.

The Diploma materials were originally printed in a similar way but this format was subsequently abandoned for two reasons. *First,* although individual Diploma blocks are offered for sale, the numbers sold are not large and the main consumers are therefore students on the Diploma course. Hence, the high cost of printing was not justified by the numbers involved. *Second,* printed materials are usually designed for a 4-5 year shelf life and can only be updated by the use of errata slips or supplements. While this is not enormously important for academic work as concepts do not change that rapidly, it can be de-motivating for students to realise that the teachers are speaking to them from 4-5 years ago. The original solution (for the Diploma) was to produce a 'Workfile' to be sent to students with their printed materials. The Workfile would be updated each year and could include the sort of informal comment or note that one would not want to print, particularly in blocks which were on general sale. Both problems were solved by the advent of 'user-friendly' desk-top publishing. These publishing systems – the DLC system is based on the 'Pagemaker' software, using an Apple Macintosh configuration with a laser printer, but there are others – have revolutionised the quality which can be obtained by in-house computer generated camera-ready copy. The internally produced pages, which were designed by an external consultant, are photocopied in small runs of several hundred in-house and spiral bound. Preliminary feedback suggests that this revised mode of producing blocks is just as acceptable to the students as the earlier printed blocks; in fact, the binding now used appears to be preferred. These materials can be produced in-house for less than half the price of printed blocks. Desk-top publishing must open up many valuable opportunities to small projects striving to produce quality learning materials that are economically viable. If such systems had been available two or three years earlier, the DLC would have avoided many problems and much expense.

Administration

Computers are also essential for the administration of the DLC. Obviously they are an enormous help in the day to day running of a busy office but there are two other crucial roles. *First,* they are potentially vital to the student record system. The Open University, for example, has always invested heavily in computer based systems and this is reflected in the existence of a separate unit – the Management Services Division – within the organisational structure of the University. Specialist software to deal with student records was designed for the DLC but to date it has not been needed, partly because the number of students – as distinct from customers – is not too large to handle with a manual system, and partly because the Polytechnic has itself moved over to a computer based student record system which can handle the current needs. We cannot yet see what the requirements for the future may be, but if the numbers of students increases it will almost certainly require additional investment in computer systems. *Second,* computers are vital for customer records. Once customer numbers are in the thousands rather than the hundreds – and that happened before the first pack was actually available – a manual system is inadequate. However, a system powerful enough to provide the sort of information on customers which is required, such as is used by mailing houses, is very expensive.

The future

Despite all the problems the DLC has, against all the odds, survived to tell the tale. In 1988 it was awarded new contracts to run along side the existing programmes. However, it seems to be increasingly clear that to establish the DLC on a sound and permanent footing requires changes in the external rather than the internal context. Quoting again from the position paper prepared in 1986:

> While the potential for generating income in the health care training market is very large, it is clear that certain constraints operate to reduce this potential:

- almost all student fees charged by institutions in higher education and the university sector are subsidised... DLC fee levels must remain competitive with these.
- external contracts rarely include a budget for any items not directly related to materials production, for example, staff development.
- similarly, external subsidy tends to be focused on particular activities...

The danger is that these constraints, acting on the DLC budget, will eventually skew the activities of the Centre in particular directions unrelated to the planned goals of the Centre... a reliance on external contracts could inhibit any staff development and would certainly curtail the broader educational and research functions concerning open learning.

Robinson 1986

Many of the Open Tech projects experienced difficulties once the subsidy from the MSC was withdrawn, not because they weren't cost effective and efficient units, but because they were competing against subsidised education. Those who criticise the open learning sector for high prices against conventional provision are not comparing like with like. However, since the extensive reorganisation of both higher education and the university sector, it is likely that the funding situation will change.

Conclusion

By reflecting on the experience of a single project we have sought to address some of the key issues of open learning. The real challenge for any production system is to be able to produce highly flexible materials that meet the diverse learning needs of the target audience. Open learning will only be cost-effective if the materials are relevant and accessible to large numbers of individuals. As Rumble (1986) remarks 'Ultimately there is no single right or wrong way of planning and managing a distance education system'. What is most important is adaptability and responsiveness to new initiatives and technological developments. Our experience has clearly shown that a small team of academics, production and administrative staff can successfully develop a range of learning materials, although it does require a great deal of hard work from everyone to do so. Like Webberley (1988), writing about his experiences of directing another Open Tech project, we too feel that we operate very close to the consequences of our own actions and that risk and responsibility are the two key factors which bind the project together.

However, only part of the success of any venture can come from within, another key element is the external context.

Acknowledgement

This chapter is based on the hard-won experience of a small team of people at the DLC which they have freely shared with us.

References

Distance Learning Centre 1986 *Teaching Patients and Clients* Managing Care Pack 9, Distance Learning Centre, South Bank Polytechnic

Lewis R and Paine N 1986 *How to Communicate with the Learner* Council for Educational Technology, Open Learning Guide 6.

Robinson K S M 1986 The Distance Learning Centre: the next five years. Unpublished paper November 1986.

Robinson K S M 1988 The distance learning mode Diploma in Nursing: a case study of collaboration, *International Journal of Nursing Studies* 25, 4, pp271-7

Rowntree D 1986 *Teaching Through Self-Instruction: a practical handbook for course developers.* Kogan Page

Rumble G 1986 *The Planning and Management of Distance Education.* Croom Helm

Webberley R 1988 Working in an Open Tech Project and the Open University: some reflections, *Open Learning* 3, 3, pp38-42

5 TASC analysis: designing and testing an open learning package

John Paley

I'm going to tell it like it is, or was.

During the last three years, and partly as a result of my experience as a project manager, I have lost all interest in the kind of writing that beats as it sweeps as it cleans. It slices off the loose ends, slaps polyfilla into the cracks, and corsets the unsightly bulges - just for the sake of a few creaky generalisations. I can't translate what happened to me into 'knowledge' that someone else can 'apply'. All I've got is a narrative - complete with mistakes, false starts, and a lot of worry. You are welcome to make sense of it if you can. It lacks only the love interest...

The chapter is 'about' designing and testing open learning material. This means that the narrative must be selective. Lots of interesting stuff will get left out, though I will need to sketch in some of the background. However, note the inverted commas: 'about'. This isn't an academic paper. It's a bit of my life, contoured.

It still happens. I'm given a topic for a study day, and turn up to find some familiar faces doing their stint as well. We all have our titles, a subject to instruct you on. But it's obvious that, in the end, they're trying to sell you their open learning package, and I'm trying to sell you mine. So perhaps I won't just be telling a story, after all. I shall also be trying to sell something. Discreetly.

The pack is called *Thinking About Social Care (TASC)*, and it's very good. It's marketed by Scroll (Social Care Open Learning Ltd.). Buy it.

The phone rang

The phone rang one day in February 1985. It was Open Tech. They had some money: did I want it? I said yes (a reflex). Great, but could I get the proposal in by tomorrow teatime? Well quickly, anyway. I knew nothing about open learning, and not much about social care. But I had spotted (with help) a gap in the market, talked to CCETSW

(Central Council for Education and Training in Social Work) and sent an outline to Open Tech. That had been about a year earlier. I'd almost forgotten.

Good news travels fast. No sooner had the Open Tech money been agreed than a delegation from Cassio College arrived at Cranfield with offers of help. They were teaching CSS (Certificate in Social Services) and ICSC (In-Service Course in Social Care) courses, to which social care staff from seventeen different agencies were regularly seconded, and they were confident that some of these agencies would be keen to take part in developmental testing. Useful. Perhaps they could also contribute to the writing? Good idea. Well, then, suppose we second some of our lecturers to the project on a part-time basis, with Scroll covering the costs of replacement? Okay, why not?

Was this arrangement a good idea? Later, I was to go through a phase of thinking it wasn't - and it probably isn't if you know what you're doing. But I didn't. Much better to commission writing on a fee basis, from people you can trust to do the kind of job you want doing. But for me, then, it was (I think now) the best option. It gave me a chance to feel my way into, and around, social care work with a group of experienced and good humoured people - whom I could meet regularly, and who didn't mind me asking stupid questions. It's difficult to do that if you have someone writing a unit in Plymouth, and somebody else writing another unit in Aberdeen. (On a subsequent project I employed a professional writer who, inconveniently, moved to Glasgow.) From a design point of view, the success of TASC owes a lot to the fortuitous creation of this team. Financially, though, it was almost certainly an error; and writing skills in the Cassio group proved to be unevenly distributed.

The brief

The brief I had inherited from the three-way discussion between Open Tech, CCETSW and Cranfield was ambitious but somewhat vague. It said that Scroll would design material focussing on attitudes - to the job, to the client, and to oneself (and other social care staff). In fact, this was one of the things that had attracted Open Tech: the challenge of designing a pack that would 'change attitudes' rather than convey knowledge and teach skills (perhaps that should read: 'in addition to' conveying knowledge and teaching skills).

Where did this brief come from? It was a natural consequence of the view, taken by CCETSW, that the pack should be suitable for 'direct care workers in the personal social services', irrespective of 'client group' and also irrespective of setting. This covers everything from children's homes to day centres for elderly people, via home helps and hostels for mentally handicapped teenagers. So the pack would have to concentrate on aspects of social care work which are common to all of these. That meant basic concepts, things like independence and self-determination for the 'client', self-awareness and 'non-judgmental' understanding for the worker. Basic, crucial, fundamental... woolly.

At least, I think that's how I saw it at the time. It's difficult to remember now. What's important is this: the concepts underlying the pack evolved. They evolved, not just by talking to the wise and good, but by writing and testing. I didn't set off with clear aims, strong ideas and well-defined objectives. I worked out what I was trying to do by trying to do it.

This may not be how you're supposed to do it. I think the more usual recommendation is that you clarify your aims, define your objectives, and then devise ways and means of fulfilling them. Temperamentally, I would have found this difficult. So I thought of something to say that would justify my approach. Fortunately, I still half believe the theory I came up with. Briefly, this says that open learning is still an experiment. We are experimenting with the concept of learner autonomy. **Q.** What does the technology of open and distance learning permit us to do that we haven't done before? **A.** Don't know, but let's try to find out. **Q.** How far can we transfer control of the learning process to the learner? **A.** Don't know, but let's see how far we can go. I have written this all up at greater length elsewhere.

The theory allowed me to argue that designing an open learning package was not something you could do *before* you started to write it. It had to be possible for experiments with technology and autonomy to change your ideas about content, structure and style as you went along. And if you didn't let this happen, all you'd end up with would be some old (rather boring) ideas about what to do and how to do it grafted on to something that should be new and exciting. It's true this argument did not convince everybody, but it kept them thinking long enough for me to change the subject and move on.

If necessary, I could always quote Nick Fox, of Open Tech, who used to say: 'Writing open learning material is not just working up your old lecture notes' - and pretend that what I said was only what he meant.

The illusion

When I'm trying to clarify something, I often succumb to the illusion that there must be a coherent, well-defined concept out there somewhere, if only I knew where to look. Someone who has a degree in philosophy shouldn't fall for that one? Okay, so I forget.

As long as you're prey to the illusion, you assume that everything you hear from the people you consult will add up to something logical and consistent. Slowly it begins to dawn on you that the reverse is the truth. Not only are people saying different things, they are actually contradicting one other. Suddenly you realise you are on a hiding to nothing. You have to make sense of it all somehow; but if you try to take account of everything that's said to you - design as the lowest common denominator - you're bound to disappoint almost everybody.

They want it in text, they want audio, they want videos, they want it computerised, they want it in braille. They want assessment, they don't want assessment (they'll assess it themselves). They want managers to supervise it, they don't want managers to supervise it. Some of them, I'll swear, want to embarrass managers with it. They want it as an alternative to ICSC. Something they do agree about is this: they want it cheap.

I can't remember precisely when the word 'flexible' started to buzz around in my head.

Dramatis personae

Who is 'they'? Let me introduce the dramatis personae. I talked to training boards, institutes, professional associations, and the like. They were - all of them - friendly, encouraging and helpful. But I never seemed to come away with more than half a page of notes. Their main concerns were not questions of design. They were more interested in the politics, which is I suppose what they're there for. This is not, emphatically, a criticism. In fact, I wish I had listened harder to some of the things I was told then. But I was looking for ideas about design, and tended to screen out everything else. I thought it amusing that someone could spend the best part of an hour ruminating on the exact significance of the word 'alternative', as in the phrase 'alternative to ICSC'. But he had a point.

I talked to training officers. They were a good source of ideas, but also a good source of contradictions. Most of them liked the concept, but each of them saw it fitting into the agency training strategy in a different way. A key issue was the degree of tutorial support that would be required. One view was: 'If you're talking about something that's going to change attitudes, how can you possibly do that without a lot of group work? I don't think I'd find it credible otherwise.' At the other end of the spectrum, someone might say: 'I've been along to sessions on other open learning packages, and they tell you it's for people working on their own. But it turns out you need a weekly group to support it. We do that already. Can't we have something a bit more self-contained?' Both of them are potential customers, the people who authorise purchase. How do I keep them both happy?

I talked to social care staff. In one crucial respect, these were the most productive conversations I had. They gave me some initial ideas about what should go into the pack - the 'content' and the 'methods'. One thing in particular struck me as being very important. Some of the staff I spoke to had been on courses of one sort or another, and I made a point of asking what had been the most useful, instructive or illuminating part of their experience. I must have put this question to over a hundred people, and I only ever got one answer that referred to something academic (it was Maslow's hierarchy of need, if anyone's interested). Almost everyone else spoke about the value of talking to other social care workers. This had to do with sharing experience; the consolation of finding other people in the same boat; and hearing 'how other people do it' and thinking 'why don't we try that?'. There seemed to be more learning going on in the comparison of 'what happens to me' and 'what happens to you' than in any number of seminars, books and articles.

Another common theme was equally interesting. It was the light shed on social care work by personal events and circumstances. There were lots of references to occasions when something happened at home which gave new meaning to a situation at work (or an idea first encountered on a course). Personal experience made something which was initially abstract or puzzling more intelligible.

At first, I wasn't sure what to do with either of these observations. But it was clear we had to avoid didacticism. Later, we decided to include stories told by social care workers - one booklet consisted of nothing else. We also decided to keep the learners active: thinking, feeling, responding, remembering, predicting, wondering, questioning.

Here's another theory. I think that research on how people learn to do their jobs - learn how to do them well or better - is at least as important as 'identifying training needs'. There are several reasons for this. One is that if you identify a need you identify a gap - but you don't necessarily get any closer to knowing how to fill it. On the other hand, if you can pinpoint an experience which various people have had, and which has led some of them to a deeper and more rounded understanding of what they do, you've got something that is altogether more positive. How did you get to be good at your job? How did you acquire the skills, the wisdom, the working knowledge? And if we put the same question to a few other people in the same business, would we get roughly the same answers? If we did, wouldn't we then have some rather strong ideas about how to encourage, accelerate and enhance the same kind of understanding in others?

This line of thought implies that we could collect lots of examples of people learning how to perform skilfully, and analyse them. We would look for these examples wherever they are to be found. You can find some of them, naturally enough, on training courses. Others you will find at the workplace, and others again in personal and domestic life. Learning can happen at any place, at any time, and it would be really interesting to know what sorts of circumstances promote what sorts of learning. So this is research - not on 'training needs' - but on how people actually learn.

And a second reason. If you set out to 'identify the training needs' of social care staff, there's an implication that you know more about the job than they do. If you're a manager or trainer, you may well feel justified in believing this - after all, you may even have drawn up the job-spec. But knowing what a job entails should be more of a dialogue. The people who do it, especially the people who learn to do it well, acquire an understanding of it that others don't - and can't - have. They understand its nuances, its rewards, its pitfalls, its possibilities. In the debate about what 'doing the job well' *means*, they have something to say which is as important as the manager's, or the trainer's, contribution. So starting from their experience, and asking what, for them, counts as 'expertise' (and how they came by it) enters into the spirit of dialogue. Just 'identifying training needs' - and leaving it at that - risks leaving something vital out.

It would be nice to think this was the sort of dialogue I was engaged in. At any rate, it was obviously a good idea to invite a small group of social care workers to join the writing team, and three students on the ICSC course at Cassio volunteered to do so.

Snap, crackle and pop?

'Make it move. Make it crackle. Make it fun. Make people *want* to use it.' It's no effort recalling the words of Edith Carpenter, the Principal Training Officer in Brent (she died, tragically, two years ago). They became axiomatic. Something I should try to explain.

Sitting here, looking at what I have just written, I think: why *did* this become so important? The honest answer is: it just appealed to me. Edith had a vision, and an enthusiasm, which rang bells. 'That's it,' I thought, 'that's something I'd like to have a go at.' There's nothing particularly logical about it. It wasn't based on an analysis of needs or markets - not an analysis I'd ever done, anyway - but it struck a chord. It would help me to feel that we were trying to be a bit different, which is good for the ego (and morale). If it worked, it might give the pack an identity of its own. And it might make the whole process of writing more enjoyable.

There is no connection between this and the conversations I had with social care staff. We are talking about two independent ideas. I did try to think of a connection (I like things tied together) but, in the end, fudged it. I also tried to think of reasons which would justify doing it that way, this time with more success. It's a question of motivation (I said). If people are going to do a course more or less on their own, and possibly with very little support from their agency, the material is going to have to hold them. Many social care workers do not have much of an academic background, and may be deterred by a pack that does not make every effort to be user-friendly. If I can quote myself at this point:

'There must be ways of making the material more attractive, of making it something that whets the appetite - something that holds, amuses, entertains and grips instead of something that bores, frustrates and deters. Naturally, this is a challenge, and to meet it we will need to divest ourselves of other sombre assumptions about education. Take humour, for instance. Humour can be highly instructive - if, once you stop laughing, you start thinking. Other genres can also be plundered for motivating colour: the thriller, the whodunnit, the strip cartoon, satire, dialogue, games, puzzles. Why should other art forms have all the best techniques? Why do education and training get left, all too often, with the horror story?'

This is me going over the top, but I still like the basic idea. But notice how it works. I didn't start with the theory and arrive at a conclusion. I started with a conclusion that appealed to me for other reasons, and worked back to the theory. Notice another implication: the justification presupposes that students will not get much support (or, at least, that the pack will have to be written on the assumption that many of them won't). So the argument means that I have to start thinking in those terms - and find ways of justifying that conclusion too.

This wasn't hard: I might well have decided to assume minimal tutorial support in any case. It was the only way of reconciling the different messages coming from training officers. Make it possible, as a bottom line, for people to do the pack virtually unsupported, and then any help they do get is a bonus. However, the fact that the backwards-working argument I have just outlined required this as a premise more or less settled matters. And that argument, you will recall, started with something that was essentially a matter of personal preference.

If all of this sounds messy, good. That's the way it was.

Content, structure, style - or style, structure, content?

I referred earlier to 'content, structure and style'. This is a handy three-way distinction, but it makes more sense in retrospect than it did at the time. On the face of it, content should come first, and you choose a structure to fit it. Content - or structure - may also determine a style, although there is more room here, presumably, for individual expression. However, it should be evident from what I've said so far, that it didn't work like that. From the consultations I had been involved in, I was getting some vague ideas - nothing more - about content, mainly from social care staff. But questions of style and structure were assuming equal, if not greater, importance. I spent more time thinking about what the pack should look like, sound like, feel like, than I did thinking about what it should actually have in it. I would not go so far as to say style and structure determined content, but there was certainly an element of that. It was not so much a matter of deciding what to do, and then finding a way of doing it. It was more like having a sense of the *how,* and then searching for a *what* that could be fitted to it.

Games, puzzles, kits, experiments, quizzes...

Picture, then, the scene at an early meeting of the writing team. We have before us a remit from Open Tech which, for some reason, we have not tried to fill out. We keep avoiding that one. I say things like: it has to be active, it has to be fun, it has to be experiential. So let's look at what we can get them to do. We all make suggestions: ideas for games, puzzles, projects, exercises, experiments, kits and quizzes. Some of the suggestions are a bit wild, some are just silly. But they all get written down (later, the ICSC students will weed out the more outrageous proposals; but they will also show enthusiasm for ideas that we, the writers, think are overboard, and say: why not try them anyway?).

Some ideas are attractive for no better reason than the fact that they seem slightly risque. For example, someone says: 'how about a fantasy role-playing game, you know like the dungeons and dragons books?' This goes down well with everybody, even though at the time we have no idea how to use it. Others are exercises which have been successful with ICSC groups. We make a note of those, too, even if we're not too sure whether they can be made to work in an open learning context.

Concepts

That's one stream. Eventually, we get round to the other: how do we tackle the 'basic' (but rather vague) concepts in the remit? This is an interesting one. Over the next few months, we keep a list of possible themes or 'topics'. What they have in common is that they are all, arguably, examples of the 'attitudes' which are referred to by the remit. Ideas are continually added to the list, while others are deleted from it. This is our 'syllabus', if anything is. We try to keep the themes in order, and the order reflects how confident we are about them - 'confident' in the sense that we are fairly sure that something of that kind ought to be included. Occasionally, we review the entire list and ask ourselves: is there any logic in this? Is there any pattern?

Again, this may seem back to front. Shouldn't the overall concept, the underlying idea, the logic, the pattern (choose your own metaphor) come first? Well, perhaps it should; but I can only tell you how it worked for us. Try this: there was a sort of circular movement; we had a few concrete ideas, and started work on them. Some of these ideas proved successful, and that gave us a certain confidence. We could then look at the whole list, bearing in mind what seemed to be working. That might suggest a more general perspective - a feel for what the 'underlying idea' might turn out to be. In turn, thoughts about this - about the general direction we seemed to be moving in - might give rise to new suggestions, which could be added to the list, or reasons why something which was already on it should be taken off.

The issue wasn't finally resolved until very late in the day, and then other considerations started to intrude. Like symmetry. For example, if we were looking at approximately sixteen booklets (we still did not know exactly how many), and if we were thinking we might want to group them into, say, four sets, wouldn't four sets of four be the best - or at least an aesthetically pleasing - way of doing it? In which case, what does it make sense to do with the remaining themes? Which should we keep in - because they would fit that pattern - and which should we leave out?

I have here smuggled in the fact that, at some point, we decided on a collection of short booklets. I'll come back to that.

Meanwhile there is an obvious question. If there were two lists, one consisting of 'how' ideas, another consisting of 'what' ideas, how did they get matched up? There's no general answer to this. It just happened. Sometimes, one of us would say: 'I fancy having a go at this topic. Which of the exercises might suit it?' Or someone would say: 'I like the idea of writing up that exercise. Which is the best theme to adapt it to?' More often, it was fortuitous. I cannot, for example, remember how the 'fantasy role-play' idea came to be hooked up to the theme of 'client autonomy' - how we came to decide on a game in which the player takes the role of an elderly person buffeted about by other people's (professional) decisions. No matter. It was a good choice. The experience of total frustration and anger that it induces in the player is precisely the point we were trying to make.

I mentioned symmetry as a fairly arbitrary consideration which began to take over later on. Another, equally arbitrary, criterion was: we began to dislike the thought of repeating ourselves. The list of 'how' ideas was quite a long one, and the first few booklets we wrote were all different. So this became a matter of honour, at least for me. I didn't want to do the same thing twice. Rationally, this is a crazy position to take - and it's fortunate that I didn't let it take over completely. But it's another interesting example of how these contingencies - matters of personal taste, personal temperament, and personal obsession - insist on having their own way.

A testing time

After a while, we had produced about half a dozen first drafts, dot matrixed, spiral bound. Ivan Gray, who was seconded from Cassio half time, had a knack of coming up with striking and/or amusing covers (he was also extraordinarily good at cartoons), so they looked interesting and reasonably presentable. Now, though, we had to test them.

We had set up a coordinating committee consisting of representatives from the Cassio team, plus training officers from the agencies which had agreed to take part in developmental testing. Their job was to recruit suitable volunteers, organise meetings, ensure that managers would cooperate, and do any other necessary ground work.

They did not all take the same view about the prospects for open and distance learning in a social care context. Although most of them were optimistic, at least one, Denis Piper, was an out-and-out sceptic - and made no bones about it. This was actually rather useful, as he asked a lot of good questions, and signalled the areas of concern and ambiguity. It was more difficult to be vague with him around. It was interesting, though, that his scepticism did not prevent him being efficient, even enthusiastic, about organising tests. His attitude seemed to me exactly the right one - open-mindedness, and a willingness to experiment. 'Even if it doesn't work, we'll have learned something. And, you never know, it might even work.' Denis deserves a mention because, as we shall see, his attitude contrasted sharply with that of some other sceptics.

We were looking for a range of people. We wanted some who had little or no experience of training, and not much experience of social care, either. This was the group for whom the pack was ultimately intended. We also wanted some with a bit more experience, people who had perhaps attended an in-service course or two, and were therefore in a position to make comparisons. When we set groups up, these were the people who were invited. In the event, however, lots of other people, including senior officers, got hold of drafts and gave us feedback. It's not giving too much away at this stage to say that most of them liked the material, whatever their background. The only significant exceptions fell into two categories. One consisted of a handful of graduate care workers (I'm not sure how or why it fell into their hands - it's not surprising that they weren't keen). The other category I'll come to later.

Each group of volunteers was asked to spend some time (usually about a month) with a batch of draft booklets (usually four). Our approach to the writing meant that, as a rule, these booklets had no obvious link with each other, and this was something that had to be explained and apologised for. The booklets were also unfinished, quite literally, so that had to be accounted for as well. Eventually, I settled into a routine and developed a workable patter.

I would visit the agency at least once, and normally twice, to explain about open learning generally and Scroll in particular. I would do a session that would spiral gradually in to what we were asking them to do, and invite comments and questions. I found people a bit difficult to warm up at first, but they tended to get more enthusiastic once the idea of open learning had sunk in. It was emphasised throughout that being present at this meeting did not imply a commitment to attending another, or to volunteering.

At a subsequent meeting, I would take a batch of material and do some more explaining. Finally, they would take the stuff away with them, sometimes taking an extra pack, if one was available, for a friend or colleague.

What I said by way of explanation is probably worth recording. The volunteers were not (I said) guinea pigs (though the idea of being a guinea pig quite appealed to many of them). They were being asked to read through the material, do the exercises, and see if they thought the ideas 'worked' or not. For anyone who felt so inclined, they were also being invited to come up with some ideas of their own, where they felt the booklets were weak or needed changing. I stressed that this was not a requirement - it was okay to write 'rubbish' on something if that was how they felt. But they would understand if I said that some sort of explanation of why it was rubbish - or suggestions as to how the offending passages could be improved - would be even more helpful.

I warned them about the weaknesses we were already aware of. I said that we were only testing out ideas and possibilities, so the drafts they would be looking at were rough and ready. There was clearly no point in doing a lot more work on something if it was going to turn out that the basic idea was no good.

For instance (I said) some of the stuff may not seem directly relevant to your own job: the examples may refer to another 'client group', or it may seem that we're just talking about residential settings and not day care, or vice versa. Things like that. This is not entirely an oversight. We do want to make it more widely relevant later, but for now we'd just like you to play with the ideas and see what you think. If something doesn't apply to you, it would be useful to know whether you think it could be adapted - and how.

Similarly (I continued) we had not always hammered out the *point* of an exercise, or even a whole booklet. This, too, was not necessarily an oversight. We were just testing ideas and wanted to know how people reacted. What did they think the point was? What, if anything, did they get out of it? Were there meanings in some of the material that we might not have noticed, might not have intended to put there? It was important that we should understand what they understood by it - so, as before, rather than just give us 'marks out of ten', some sort of commentary would be very much appreciated.

We were also asking them to keep an eye on such things as humour (did it sometimes go over the top? Was it always relevant?) as well as on presentation and style. The 'feel' of material - was it (as we hoped) accessible and entertaining, or was it just forced, silly, irritating?

In conclusion, we were inviting them to be, in effect, co-authors. I did not want to patronise them by exaggerating this but, nevertheless, their contribution was vital. No-one should feel obliged to respond to this part of the invitation; but anyone who wished to do so could feel confident that what they had to say would be taken into account in the final version - allowing for inevitable differences of opinion.

I obviously don't want to go into the feedback in detail, showing you all the best bits. The main point is that a significant proportion of volunteers took the invitation seriously, and that what they said not only helped us to re-write the booklets, but also forced us to revise some of our ideas about the pack as a whole. The volunteers, in this sense, participated fully in the design.

I'll give some examples of this in a moment. First, though, I want to take a short but interesting detour.

Into trouble

Somewhere in all this I was starting to get into trouble: 'Dear Sir, I am rather worried about what he is getting up to.' Letters of this kind, but longer, were being despatched to Open Tech by members of my advisory group. I have not mentioned this group yet, mainly because it was dormant during the first few months of the project.

Background: It was a condition of the contract that a steering group be set up. Before the project began, I took advice from CCETSW as to its compostion; but after nearly eight months there had still not been a meeting, the problem being that I could get no response from the ADSS (Association of Directors of Social Services), which CCETSW strongly advised should be represented. On previous occasions, and in regard to other ventures, the ADSS had sent me snappy two-liners bordering on discourtesy; but no letter at all was a departure. In the end, I went ahead without them.

Despite the contract, the steering group did not have a constitution and, when it finally got together, the project had been under way for some little time. On top of this, TASC was not intended to be part of qualifying training, nor was it a supplement to any other validated programme - so there was little scope for comment on how far it did or did not conform to validation requirements. As a result, the steering group spent a lot of time fretting about its 'role'. My own doubts about this prompted me to refer to the group as 'advisory' rather than 'steering'.

By all accounts, I was not the only project manager who had a rather tense relationship with her/his steering/advisory group, and it's in the nature of things, probably, that these tensions should exist. But let me offer a synopsis of what I think the source of the trouble was, in my case. This, I should add, with the benefit of hindsight.

Craft, or science?

There's a bit of a contradiction. Open Tech projects had to serve an immediate need, and they had to be marketable. Your admiration for 'market forces' does not have to be total (mine isn't). It's still possible to believe that what's needed, what works, what people think it would be nice to have, what (in the end) they are willing to invest in, are important considerations. Looking back, this has something to do with what I've already said about experiment and dialogue, and with a certain pragmatic, suck-it-and-see approach to producing material.

But there is another set of considerations which, sometimes, may come into conflict with the first set. These are the 'doing it properly' considerations. Training is one of those areas in which an enormous amount of experience has generated an enormous amount of literature on how to get it right. A lot of this literature is very valuable, as it could hardly fail to be, given the history of trial and error that lies behind it. Like any literature, it can be treated as a collection of handy tips, rules of thumb, accounts of things that have been known to work and might just work again.

Unfortunately, however, there is a tendency to overdo it. Rules of thumb become algorithms and paradigms, interesting narratives become theory. The whole thing is made to look far more rational, and more 'scientific', than it really is. This is, partly at least, the fault of the academic genre we all have to write in, derived from scientific journals, crammed with footnotes and references (though it's also got something to do with theories about management, which is equally prone to tarting itself up as a science).

There is a clash - there was a clash - between the academic standpoint and the more freewheeling 'let's just try this and see if it works...' I only have myself to blame. Members of the advisory group inspected my reports - and the first draft booklets - for things like learning objectives, statements of competencies (as they are now called), task and/or job analysis, the derivation of training needs, and criteria of evaluation. They looked in vain. They had qualms. They wrote to Open Tech. They were worried that I did not know what I was doing.

They were right. In one sense, I did not (yet) know what I was doing. I had no overall concept, no objectives, no firm sense of direction. I had nothing but a lot of interesting ideas (mainly other people's), and some very encouraging feedback from social care staff and training officers. The volunteers understood that they were taking part in an experiment. The advisory group had some difficulty with that. The volunteers did not mind the absence of learning objectives. They were keen to tell us what they had got out of the booklets they had worked with, and to make practical suggestions as to how the exercises could be improved. They took it as read that the final, published, version of the booklets would look very different from the first drafts. The advisory group had some trouble with that, too.

It was my own fault. I could have explained what was going on better than I did. But I lost patience with unnecessary abstraction (which is how I saw it), and the steering/advisory group's indifferences to the response from the field (which is how I interpreted it). However, Open Tech was threatening to withhold some cash, so I wrote a rather whining 'response to criticism', and managed to keep the show on the road. But here's a thought. Suppose the experiment hadn't worked... Experiments still have to be paid for. All that public money gone up in smoke? So wasn't the advisory group right to be worried about my cavalier attitude? I think they probably were. But when, towards the end of the project, one of the more sympathetic members of the group described it as a millstone round my neck, I didn't think. I just nodded.

How many of these things are there going to be?

'How many of these are there going to be?', asked one volunteer, quite early on. She was referring to the booklets. It was a question which re-framed my thinking about the structure of TASC. Up to then, we had left open the matter of how the pack would be organised, assuming that at some point our jig-saw pieces would show us a coherent picture and that one bit would lead to another bit, and then to another. This one question triggered a completely different line of thought.

Suppose that, instead of fitting the themes into a framework, we built the framework round a collection of themes? It was obvious, when you saw it, and certainly consistent with how we'd done things up to now. Each theme would be explored in two or three exercises - as strong and colourful as we could make them - and that would constitute a booklet. The pack would just be a series of these booklets.

And the answer to the next question arrived before the question itself did. The answer was: you wouldn't need to do them in any particular order, would you? The question was: what order should the booklets come in? The answer was *very* interesting, because it meant there was something an open learning pack could do that an in-service course couldn't, as a rule - have the students all doing different parts of the course at the same time. And that meant the students could choose an order to suit them. What factors might influence the choice? They might do a booklet just because it looked interesting. Or they might do it because another booklet referred to it, and it seemed a logical step (which meant there would have to be plenty of cross-references). Or they might do it because it dealt with something that was happening at work, and so was particularly relevant at the time. All sorts of possibilities.

That led to another question. You've got a collection of booklets, and it's an attractive option to let people work through them in any order. How do you make sense of that in terms of an overall concept, an 'underlying idea'? Because you can't have later booklets relying - building - on earlier ones. There won't *be* earlier and later ones that are the same for everybody. Okay, let's have a look at the list of themes. Does that help? Well, there's something implicit in it that might. See them all as different facets of a single topic - the central, crucial, fundamental topic of the relationship between the social care worker and the 'client'. (There may be a problem about the ones we've already done on team work. But even that makes sense, when you think about it, and in any case I can worry about it later.)

So the booklets will all be about the same thing, in effect? But they will come at it from a number of different angles, using a variety of different methods. It will be like trying to create a new gestalt, a way of seeing and understanding that encompasses the themes built into each booklet. Come at the same basic idea in a range of guises, and with a slightly different perspective each time, and sooner or later (we hope) the penny will drop. Gosh! Holistic learning! (But don't get into the habit of using *that* expression, for heaven's sake.)

There are more questions, more loose ends. Like: what does this tell us about what else needs to be on the list of themes - or on the list of exercises? And so on, round the circle. I won't develop it all. I've just tried to outline the first rush of thinking...

All that from a single question posed by this volunteer. And still I haven't answered *that* question: How many booklets will there be?

I probably don't need to labour the point again. A crucial part of the answer to the question, 'What exactly are we trying to do?', did not turn up until we had started to write and test the first drafts. And everything hung on a contribution from one of the volunteers.

Thinking about social care

By way of a conclusion, let me rattle through a few more examples of design issues that were raised, or resolved, through testing. They are in no particular order.

I had imagined that most people would struggle through the booklets on their own (if I'd thought about it at all). Admittedly, some of the exercises required a partner - two-player games, for example. But I thought people would grab a passing colleague, perhaps a friend or a member of the family. What I did not bargain for was the way in which some volunteers paired off for the duration, and did all the booklets together. Without fail, the people who had done this always seemed to have got the most out of it, always seemed to have most to say about it - often had the most thoughtful comments to make. This was so impressive and so consistent a feature of the tesing that we began to take account of it in drafting subsequent booklets. While it is still possible for people to work on their own - with occasional help - the learners are encouraged to pair off, and the published version of the pack is full of references to 'your Scroll partner'.

I was also amazed by the range of people who had got hold of a copy, and who turned up to review meetings (not having attended the earlier ones). This was undoubtedly thanks to the humour, which made all the booklets very mobile. They were passed round, photocopied, cartoons were stuck on walls and notice boards. This got people interested. Groups were formed, sometimes a senior officer got involved. Some booklets had been used in team discussion, study days and supervision. Some of the pencil-and-paper exercises were being used for regular monitoring.

This isn't just boasting (well, okay, a bit). The point is that all this fed back into our thinking, and in at least two different ways. One was the number of new ideas suggested or requested. We'd like to use the supervision record sheet as a regular thing, but it would need the following modifications... Our team is using the decision-making ladder/stress scale/network maps, but we want to know if we can adapt them and, if so, how... This stuff on the uses of supervision is all very well, but what if you don't get any? Can't we have something on how to *get* supervision? And so on.

The second way was more conceptual. There are obviously multiple uses for this material, and more than one context in which people are going to do things with it. Without going mad, can we allow for that in how we draft more of it? Perhaps encourage it? But then, what can we say about 'learning objectives' (the expression was in circulation by now, following the set-to with the advisory group). Possibly that there *are* no determinate, off-the-peg objectives which must be the same for everybody? 'Here are some interesting things to do, stories to read, questions to ask, projects to carry out. They will make you think... And that's *it*. We can guess at what they might make you think about, and we can tell you that if you want to know (see the last page). But the main point is ending up somewhere different from where you started - and thinking got you there.'

Two spin-offs. Call this 'ceding control of learning objectives', and you have a nice theory about one implication of distance learning. I have written about that elsewhere. That's the first spin-off. The second is a title: *Thinking About Social Care*.

Remember to get yourself a copy.

Thinking

That would be a good way to finish, wouldn't it? But it's never that simple. A muddling through story can't end that perfectly. There's one loose end left over, and it can't be ignored: the second category of people who did not much like the draft material they saw (the first was graduates, you will recall). This was a group of Afro-Caribbeans, specifically those who had had a West Indian education. This group did not want the training they took part in to have the 'light touch' we were beginning to pride ourselves on. They wanted it to be more seriously serious. One woman complained that she had read everything twice: once to identify the jokes and cross them out, and once to get something out of the material... 'There's some interesting things in it, but you've got to get past all that irritation first.'

I wish there were more space to explore this issue, and others related to it. I am aware that I underestimated the difficulty of ensuring that the pack would be non-racist, and I am still not sure what the implications of making it anti-racist would be. In the first draft booklets, there were many places in which the issue of racism could and should have been raised, but it wasn't. They still exist in the final version, though (I think) there are fewer of them. The lesson I learned - and I was thoroughly, but gently, mauled by a small group of black workers one memorable weekend in Newport Pagnell - was that there is such a thing as racism (and indeed sexism) by default. It is possible to reinforce racist attitudes simply by not challenging them.

We tried to avoid the obvious pitfalls, and the places where we failed were brought to our attention by both black and white volunteers. We took steps to ensure that material was screened by people of several different races and cultures. But they probably weren't hard enough on us. First black worker: 'That cartoon is offensive. It ought to be changed like this...'. Second black worker: 'But then it would not be funny, and the point of it would be lost...'. This was a cartoon we removed, but ambiguities like this can easily be used as an excuse for doing not very much. Whatever else, I am certain that we have not done nearly enough.

Footnote

As you will have gathered, I wanted (for all kinds of reasons) to write something autobiographical. Packing the text with references didn't seem consistent with that. However, two essays of my own are mentioned in passing, and you might want to look them up. They are:

(i)   Open learning and vocational education: concepts and questions for the caring professions. Paper presented to a CCETSW conference in February 1986, and available from School of Policy Studies, Cranfield Institute of Technology.

(ii)   The Challenge of Open Learning *Nursing Times,* 10.12.86.

They cover roughly the same ground, though the first is much longer and more detailed.

What I would really like to do, though, is refer to *people* rather than literature, because a lot of friends and colleagues provided ideas, help and encouragement (words too, sometimes). It is to them that the real thanks is due. The only problem is knowing where to stop as the list is potentially endless. I do know that the following people all left their mark, in some crucial way, on my thinking - and, often, on the finished product: Sue Billington, David Bowdler, Edith Carpenter, Paul

Ellerington, Ivan Gray, Sue Greene, Tony Hewitt, Judith Hughes, Martyn Jones, Wilfred Lowe, Chris Paley, Chris Payne, Denis Piper, Alan Rhodes, Kate Robinson, Leo Smith, Maureen White, Hester Willson.

6 Writing for competencies

Barbara Vaughan

Nursing is basically a practice discipline and as such needs to prepare people who are competent, not only in 'knowing that' or understanding the theory which is taught, but also in 'knowing how' or being able to practice. It can be argued that a theoretical understanding alone of a subject matter which can be applied to a practice discipline does not in itself produce competent practitioners. However, the argument is equally strong that people who are skilled in 'doing' without understanding are potentially dangerous since their decisions are made from an unsound basis. Thus what is required is the mixing of the two types of competence in the 'knowledgeable doer' since 'competency is only achieved when the occupation is performed proficiently in all its aspects, ie good practice based on sound knowledge'. (Jarvis 1984). If open learning is to be a successful aid to learning for nurses then we must seek a way of using it to help people not only to deepen their understanding of the academic disciplines which underpin their work but also of exploring their own experiential knowledge and understandings of self and others and of combining all this knowledge into efficient and effective nursing actions. Open learning for nurses is therefore firmly in the arena of vocational rather than general education, but unlike other vocational educational programmes which are concerned with efficiency and effectiveness, in nursing the necessity for *humanity* in action adds a further complicating dimension of competence for the educator to deal with.

The components of nursing competence

In the early seventies the then Joint Board of Clinical Nursing Studies identified three areas in which competency was sought, namely knowledge, skills and attitudes. Jarvis (1984) suggests that these are in fact the major elements of professional competency, expanding them as:

competent they are in practical skills or whether or not their attitudes are acceptable to their chosen profession.

Acquiring competency through open learning

These descriptions of competency suggest that the goal of learning in nursing goes well beyond the mere acquisition of new theoretical knowledge to helping the practitioner to feel and *be* able to offer a better service to the client. The challenge is the same in any mode of teaching, but the writing of open learning materials seems to present the dilemmas more acutely, perhaps because the separation of teacher (author) and learner removes the frequent interaction between them and thus the possibility of making opportunistic links between the different types of knowledge in practice. These links have to be built into the text and tested again and again for validity in the developmental stages of writing. Such a challenge is not easy to face up to but there are compensations as well as difficulties in writing open learning materials. In particular, it is very helpful to know that the learner can take the learning materials into her workplace and can be asked to work through particular activities in her real context with her clients and colleagues. It has been perceptively remarked that the 'distance' label refers to the separation of teacher and learner and not the separation of the learner from her workplace which is the appropriate learning environment. Perhaps the concept 'distance' should, within vocational education, be applied to conventional teaching.

Extrapolating key issues from the comments made so far there are certain fundamental questions which have to answered by those who prepare open learning materials before the 'real work' of writing begins. In many ways they resemble the stages of any curriculum development activity but in some instances the options available may be different since a different medium is being used. These questions include:

- what is the purpose of this course?
- who is the course being prepared for?
- how will the outcomes be assessed?
- how can I help the learner achieve the aims of the course through the text?

In conventional situations there is always the option of adopting *pro tem* solutions which are sufficient as working guides; changes can then be made as the course progresses and the teachers find out what works and what does not. It is often acknowledged that the first cohort through a new course are in a sense 'guinea pigs' for testing the curriculum. However, in the open learning situation such options are not usually available; course materials are produced for a lifetime of anywhere between four and eight years and are not usually revised before then on grounds of cost. P553 *A Systematic Approach to Nursing Care* (Open University 1984) for example, was mainly written in 1983, printed in 1984 and not revised until 1989. In that time it is estimated that over 60,000 learners had used it (Liddiard 1989). An error in the writing could therefore have had major consequences.

The course team

These are complex questions and for any course a curriculum planning team would be established to produce solutions. The equivalent in open learning terms is the production course team, which is a team of people who plan and produce the course material and often see the course through the first year of use. Thereafter the course is no longer 'in production' and, although the learners obviously need support, the course itself requires only a relatively small amount of input which can be provided by a maintenance course team. The size and mix of the production course team will obviously vary according to the material under preparation but it can be said that in all cases there are three essential requirements:

- experts in the subject in hand
- representatives of the potential consumers
- someone who has experience of writing learning packs.

Experts

One of the major advantages of learning materials is that students can have access to the views and opinions of a wide range of experts which would not necessarily be so in a more traditional approach to learning. For P553 this was an important advantage as the nursing process was a relatively new introduction to the UK and expertise was very thinly spread throughout the country. The expertise assembled consisted of:

- Nursing Process Coordinator, Cambridge Health District
- Nursing Research Liaison Officer, Northern Regional Health Authority
- Adviser and Coordinator for the Nursing Process in England and Wales, DHSS
- Clinical Lecturer in Nursing, Manchester University/Ward Sister, Manchester Royal Infirmary
- Senior Nurse, Clinical Practice Development, Oxfordshire Health Authority

- Nurse Consultant, Services for the Elderly, Cambridge Health District
- Nurse academic/author
- Senior Tutor, Nursing Practice Development, Oxfordshire Health Authority.

Open University 1984

This team offered a reasonable balance between researchers, lecturers, practitioners and others, and also allowed input from various parts of the country. The combination of different types of expertise within one team is especially important in a practice discipline like nursing which draws on many applied sciences for knowledge, and it is important that the balance is right and that no one discipline of them 'takes over' from the nursing knowledge which should lie at the heart of the material.

Consumers

The P553 course team itself represented many of the potential consumers of the course, or at least those who would be using the course with learners. However, through the use of critical commentators who read and commented on draft materials this pool was expanded to include a number of post-basic tutors (Open University 1984).

Open learning expertise

The importance of retaining expertise in open learning can hardly be overestimated; in the case of P553 the Course Team Chair was based in the Institute of Educational Technology at the Open University and could guide us in the techniques and strategies to achieve our aims. If this is not possible, as may sometimes be the case, it is strongly recommended that advice is sought as the skill of writing open learning is quite different from either writing for publication or preparing more conventional lessons. However, not all open learning specialists are skilled in writing for competencies rather than abstract knowledge and it would be essential to discuss your aims with them before beginning collaborative work.

If possible it might be worth considering running a workshop for potential authors to help them gain these skills. This was the strategy when the *Nursing in Community Hospitals* learning pack was being prepared (Oxfordshire Health District/DLC forthcoming). All the authors met over a weekend with open learning specialists to develop the writing skills which are specific to learning materials, particularly the art of interacting with the learner and helping the learner interact with and learn from her environment.

The purpose of the course

Once the course planning team meet their primary task must be to clarify exactly what it is that they wish to achieve and it is surprising how much variation there is amongst people who believe themselves to be working to a common goal. For example, in the early stages of preparing P553 there was a great debate centred around two major issues. First, what knowledge was required by the practitioner to be able to use the nursing process; variations of opinion arising initially over whether there was a need to explore the nature of nursing itself. The course could have presented the nursing process as just a simple decision making and planning tool, which in one sense it is, but because the learner was being asked to use it in a *practice* situation it was set within a more general framework of other nursing competencies. In essence the course philosophy was that the learner could not be said to be competent in the *nursing* process unless she had the skills of relationship building, teamwork, using a nursing model, etc. which are essential *nursing* competencies. Of the seven 'core themes' around which the course was eventually designed, only one relates to simple problem solving skills, the others relate to wider competencies within nursing such as forming a relationship between the nurse and patient. The course team may constitute a sufficient resource to define competencies, but if not they should consult more widely. The Open University, for example, often begins the planning process for materials for professional groups with workshops to get a broad spectrum of opinion. Dunn and Hamilton (1985) suggest a number of more formal methods for exploring relevant competencies, such as task analysis, the Delphi technique, Critical Incident Survey and the Behavioural Event Interview.

The course planning team must identify how far they want learners to acquire the new types of knowledge described above and how to help them combine them in practice. When competency in nursing practice is the aim then the whole of the design of the course must be geared to activities which will help the learner to interact with his or her clinical environment.

Who is the course being prepared for?

It is difficult for the authors of open learning material to know in detail the backgrounds of the people who will be using it. There will be information about the professional qualification of the learner and the type of work environment but within these parameters there is obviously a great variety. Nursing is not a homogeneous occupation and the various branches and specialties vary enormously in the things they do and indeed in the models and philosophies they hold. A balance has to be sought between meeting the needs of those who are relatively new to the topics in question and maintaining the interest and providing stimulus for those who are experienced, and between the interests of the different specialties likely to be using the materials. However, the more the learner is invited to bring her own knowledge and experience into the materials the less of a problem this will be.

How will outcomes be assessed?

Obviously the aims of the course should be reflected in the assessment procedures, and a course which is concerned with competence should maintain that focus consistently. However, assessment can take place both within the materials and in formal procedures apart from the materials and the author may not be involved in the latter, having to work within the parameters set by others. If so, she should try to guide the learner towards the key issues and knowledge which will be assessed even if it does not entirely reflect the outcomes which she would want to emphasise, as 'mixed messages' will only serve to confuse the learner.

Within the materials the author can help the learner assess her progress through the use of devices in the text such as 'in-text questions and answers' and commentaries on learner activities, which are described in more detail below. These offer an immediate response to the learner who has some reassurance that she is 'on the right lines'. In some instances the feedback may be limited to a debate about the complexity of the question with a few comments of the author's. Indeed in many cases there is no right or wrong answer, a fact which many nurses find difficult to come to terms with. But if we are seeking to help people to develop as autonomous practitioners, living with uncertainty and accepting that there are times when there is not a clear cut answer itself becomes an important competence.

There are times when the learners require the reassurance of more formal feedback but not within a formal assessment system. In my experience of running P553 groups I have found it helpful to offer to work through the learners' workbooks with them on an individual basis in order to help them to assess their own progress. It is also possible to ask students to submit assignments for comment and some indication of their level of work. Although the authors of the material cannot offer this sort of face-to-face tuition, they can organise the material so that it is easy for group leaders to integrate it into the whole learning experience, and they can make sure that the competence based nature of the material is explicit. The P553 materials include group leader notes to guide them on the nature of the materials and on appropriate activities.

The formal assessment of practice based open learning at post-registration level is likely to become more common in the future, particularly with the advent of alternative routes for enrolled nurses to

convert to registration and with the growing number of schemes such
as Health Pickup and MESOL (for a brief discussion of Health Pickup
and MESOL see Chapter 1). For such programmes it is the awarding
bodies who will make the decision as to what competencies are valued
and how they will be assessed but ideally the formal assessment system
should be integrated into the in-text informal feedback to the learner
so that she can take part in her own assessment and learn to assess
her competencies.

Producing text

Bearing in mind the ideas of the discussion above, the production of
text needs to be guided by the following principles:

- make the relevance of the learning to practice explicit at a
  very early stage;
- make use of the wealth of knowledge which the learner
  already has through professional experience and life itself;
- make it clear that what is sought is personal growth and
  collaboration with others;
- give the student a degree of control in both the timing and
  depth of study.

The great temptation when writing open learning materials is to say
'this is how to do it'; to dominate rather than facilitate. And many of
the devices available to authors of open learning texts can convey the
message of domination; listing set objectives, for example, or including
summaries of content. Within the body of the text the choice of
content is also important and should avoid prescription. In P553, for
example, we choose to include brief accounts of three different nursing
models, and while this was appropriate when models were very new
ideas, the approach neglects other important skills such as how to
choose or adapt a model for individual circumstances. The new
supplementary material for the pack therefore doesn't choose a
number of other models to include but discusses types of model and
the possibilities of choosing a model or building your own. Clinical
competency in the use of models requires a 'convergence' of the
theoretical ideas about models with the ideas about the philosophy of
nursing which emerge from practice and an exploration of one's self
and one's view on the nature of humanity and the possibilities for
change.

Similarly we tried not to 'tell' learners how to do assessments but to
help learners both understand the different frameworks which can be
used to guide nursing assessment and to make discriminating decisions
about how much data to collect in differing circumstances. Showing

competence means adjusting an assessment framework to the particular needs of individual patients or different settings.

So, although competencies are often linked to particular areas of practice, such as nursing models or health education or drug administration, the open learning author must also remember the common theme that the practitioner must be competent to *act*, and to act safely and with humanity. It is therefore important that, as well as dealing with empirical knowledge, the text encourages both reflection and self-exploration *and* practical decision making. The structure of the text will carry a great deal of this message to the learner, through a number of methods such as:

- practice exploration activities
- reflective activities
- knowledge tests
- group learning prompts
- offering alternative routes and pacing

It is important that whichever methods are chosen, they should be integral to the text, not additional extras. Many learning materials ask the learner to undertake activities at regular intervals as they progress through the text but many people find it tempting to 'skip' some of the exercises. If this happens much of the value is lost since this is the major way in which the learner has an opportunity to react to what is being discussed. This becomes even more important when clinical skills are taught since the activities are frequently geared towards practising new skills in an environment which is familiar to the learner. Thus if competencies are to be gained it is essential that the activities are interesting, relevant and varied, drawing the learner's attention from the familiar to the unfamiliar. If learners can skip the activities and still make sense of the materials then perhaps the materials are inappropriately written; if the learner's contribution is really being taken seriously then the product of the activities undertaken by the learner becomes an integral part of the course. This can be expressed by basing activities on the learner's work for a previous activity. In a sense the material is not complete until the learner has worked through it. The 'authors' of the material in this sense are both the named 'teacher' who wrote it *and* the learner.

Activities

P553 made extensive use of activity based on learning of two types –
reflective and exploratory. An example of a reflective activity can be
seen in Figure 6.1 and an example of an activity encouraging the

---

Activity 1.6   *Allow 15 minutes*

A model for you?

*You might have found the section on models contained a lot of ideas
which are new to you and which may need further thought. This activity
is intended to assist you in understanding the concept of nursing
models.*

Consider the three major elements which go towards making a model for
practice and, using the following headings, briefly outline your own ideas
about a nursing model. They may reflect those described in the text or have
arisen from other sources.

1 Beliefs about Man

2 Goals of care

3 Knowledge for practice

Authors' comment
*It is difficult to put a time limit on an activity of this kind as ideas often
emerge over a long period. However, having considered some of your
own thoughts, you may find it helpful to spend some further time
discussing and comparing them with those colleagues with whom you
work.*

Figure 6.1   Reflective activity

Activity 1.7   *Allow 5 minutes*

What are you accountable for?

*In this activity we ask you to think about your own practice in relation
to the preceding discussion.*

Think back to the last time you were working in your own area and
consider one clinical decision which you made during your span of duty, for
example the action you prescribed to prevent the formation of deep venous
thrombosis. Consider how you would defend that decision to your own peer
group and the reason why you thought that action was necessary.

Authors' comment
*We hope that your decision was grounded on research-based knowledge
rather than on tradition, routine or myth.*

Figure 6.2   Explorative activity

exploration of practice can be seen in Figure 6.2. Some activities, such
as that in Figure 6.3, combined both types. Decisions about whether
and how to construct such comments should be determined by the
aims of the course. If the aim is to allow the learner space to develop

her own thinking and ideas then it is important that they do not carry the message that there is a 'right' answer. Equally, in a situation where you cannot guarantee that the learner will have any support at all with her studies a carefully constructed comment might offer encouragement that she is thinking along similar lines to other learners or thinking at an appropriate depth. However, you do not need to have comments with every activity; for example, England (1987) usefully differentiates between 'stop and think' activities which do not carry any feedback and 'think and write' activities which do.

Activity 4.7   *Allow 10 minutes*
Getting involved with your patients
This activity aims to help you think about the practicalities of forming close relationships with your own patients and their families.
List any practical difficulties or personal anxieties which you think may occur if you get more closely involved with your patients and their families.

Authors' comment
You have probably included some or all of the following points in your list and, of course, you may have others:
- *difficulty in finding time to develop relationships*
- *patient and/or family becoming dependent on you and making demands which you can't meet*
- *difficulty in bringing the relationship to an end without one or both parties feeling a sense of loss, or feeling 'let down'*
- *fear of emotional 'drain' from being so close to a constant stream of people who all have complex needs and concerns*
- *feeling inadequately prepared to handle close relationships with patients – they may ask questions which you can't answer or express emotions that disturb you.*

Figure 6.3   Reflective and explorative activity

Describing a timing for activities may also help to encourage the learner by indicating that it wouldn't be usual to be able to answer the question in less than, say, ten or fifteen minutes. Nevertheless the tension between *description* and *prescription* is always present and it is important that the learner doesn't feel inhibited by them. For example, although each of the modules in P553 are supposed to take about four hours we know that they often take rather longer, and one learner reported taking 36 hours – but, as she was dyslexic this was obviously the right length of time for her.

Perhaps the most radical open learning materials which are being used by nurses are those of the Open University course D321 *Professional Judgment*. The course is not merely *about* making decisions, it also *consists* of making decisions. The learner is encouraged throughout the course to make decisions and judgments and to evaluate both her own judgments and those of her tutor. Learners are explicitly rewarded for admitting the limitations of their knowledge and also for the quality of their attempts rather than the quality of their achievement. The course uses a number of writing styles including dialogue between the author and an imaginary doctor. Such a course seems to offer useful precedents of style and method to authors struggling to help nurses with competencies.

Knowledge tests

These are not really exploratory activities but rather offer the learner evidence that she is coping with the text. In their simplest form they just check that the learner has understood what she has been told, but of course their usefulness will be limited in any text which sets out to facilitate learning rather than give the learner information. Nevertheless they have a number of uses such as helping the learner check she has remembered terms correctly, as in this self-assessment question :

> What term is employed to describe the attempted complete control of the state over its population in state socialist societies?
> Hughes 1987

However, if the materials are being used for a formally assessed course which does not explicitly value practice based competencies, it is important for the learner that she is given 'cues' as to what to concentrate on and what the key themes are in order that her assignment will reflect the curriculum values. While acknowledging that this may not encourage openness, it may be expedient.

Group learning prompts

These are activities which encourage the learner to enter into discussions with colleagues and peers. They are particularly useful in a situation where there is no group work built into the course, but they also help to integrate the learning experiences of the course into the learner's work environment. The following example of an activity which prompts group work is taken from a workbook for the Diploma in Nursing:

> Make a list of at least four other occupational groups with whom you work on a regular basis. For each group, answer the following questions:
> 1 What is the major goal of the service they offer?
> 2 What are the major topics included in their education and training?

3 What do you see as their contribution to patient care?
4 How do you maintain an understanding of each other's
   work?
   Having noted down your own views, check them out for
   accuracy by asking the people concerned whether or not they
   share them.

Robinson and Vaughan 1988

Alternative routes

One of the great advantages of using materials rather than a teacher is
that the learner can embark on her learning experience in any way
that she chooses. I have always suspected that many people enter
P553 via the cartoons which therefore have at least two functions –
first to illustrate a point made in the text but second to entice the
reader into the text. However, despite the possibility of multiple entry
points, few texts are designed in other than a linear fashion. The
logical progression of the text is from page one to 'the end'. Certainly
this was the case with P553 where the modules were organised to
reflect the stages of the nursing process. This in itself created a
problem because we wanted to emphasise that the process was itself
more dynamic than the steps implied:

> Although we have separated the stages of the nursing process
> for the purposes of description, in practice the whole process is
> integrated. The sequence of steps follows a spiral route rather
> than a climb up the four steps of a ladder...

Open University 1984

One way in which we could have emphasised the dynamic nature of
the process would have been to write a more complexly structured text
in which the learner had to deal with assessment, planning,
implementation and evaluation all at the same time – as one does with
a patient. However, this might present real difficulties to some of the
learners who use the pack who are both unused to studying and
unfamiliar with the ideas being introduced. So there is a tension which
has to be resolved by the authors between offering the learner a
flexible learning environment and a reasonable sense of security.
However, opting for the safety of a carefully signposted and fenced
route through the text may also cause problems for some learners as
'The student's learning path may match, conflict with or compromise
the learning path set up in the materials'. (England 1987)

The idea of a non-linear course has been explored elsewhere, however.
For example, the Social Care Open Learning Project (SCROLL 1987:
see Chapter 5) which produced a course as a series of short – about

forty pages – booklets which can be read in any order. This obviously offers the learner a flexibility and choice which the 180 linear pages of P553 do not. However, the writing of short 'chunks' of learning requires operating within very tight constraints and the author needs to be quite clear about what is to be achieved in *each* booklet as extensive cross-references and the pursuit of complex themes is just not possible within the space.

Safe practice

One of the problems of writing open learning materials which are intended to encourage practical action is that the learner and her client may be endangered in ways which we cannot predict. For example, in preparing materials on the nursing process it was suggested that an activity should centre on the learner assessing the physical status of her client. Leaving aside the question of how appropriate a nursing activity that might be, it proved impossible, within the constraints of the length of the materials, to ensure that the materials guided the learner into making it a safe and caring procedure for her client.

Similarly the learner may be put at risk by some activities. For example, the following activity is potentially dangerous:

> Look up a definition of the word 'prejudice'. What is the difference between prejudice and discrimination? Think of examples of both that you have been involved with or witnessed.

> Rafferty and Robinson 1988

Here the recollection of a disturbing event, perhaps one in which the nurse was harassed or failed to act in support of someone else may be disturbing. However, the authors knew that the materials were designed for use within a course which offered support to the learners, so it seemed a reasonable risk. In other circumstances a different decision might have been made.

There are many less dramatic examples of activities which might merely depress or frustrate the learner by asking her to, for example, contact a continuing education tutor or refer to a specialist nurse when neither was available. For these reasons the degree of openness and choice which should be included in learning materials may depend on the specification of the intended audience.

The testing of materials in the developmental stage with groups of 'typical' learners is an important part of the writing process. It tests whether the methods which have been used to help the learner are working and, at a more basic level, whether the text is intelligible at all. Particularly it should check that the authors have not slipped back into teaching theory in isolation from practice. However, it is also important that this issue of safety for the learner and her patient is addressed in developmental testing where group leaders are available to 'pick up the pieces' in a way which may not be possible once the pack is on open sale.

Conclusion

The issue of how to help nurses achieve competence in expert independent nursing practice is very much on the current agenda of nurse education. A number of important innovations have recently been introduced to ensure that learning is based in practice and oriented towards the provision of care rather than acquisition of abstract empirical knowledge. For example, the introduction of the lecturer-practitioner role (Vaughan 1989) can be seen as a vital step forward. The increased use of open learning in nurse education can be set within this movement as it can be very useful in helping nurses to gain either their basic competencies or further expertise in practice. However, this will only be the case if the authors of materials face up to the real challenge of writing for practice based competencies rather than empirical ones. Such writing is, in my experience, extremely difficult and takes a major investment of time, demanding that the author explores her own ideas about practice and competence. Nevertheless, there is within open learning for nursing the beginnings of a debate about writing for competencies in which we can explore new methods of helping learners become independent of the classroom and relate their learning to their real needs as practitioners.

References

Benner P, Wrubel J 1989 *Primacy of Caring, Stress and Coping in Health and Illness.* Addison Wesley

Downie R and Calman K 1987 *Healthy Respect: Ethics in Health Care.* Faber

Carper B 1978 Fundamental patterns of knowing in nursing, *Advances in Nursing Science.* October 1 (*v*) 13-23

Dunn W R and Hamilton D D 1985 Competence based education and distance learning: a tandem for professional continuing education? *Studies in Higher Education, 10, 3*

England E 1987 The design of versatile text materials *Open Learning, 2, 2*

Hughes G 1987 *Looking at Society.* Distance Learning Centre, South Bank Polytechnic

Jarvis P 1984 *Professional Education.* Croom Helm

Johns C, Pearson A, Robinson K S M and Vaughan B (eds.) forthcoming *Nursing in Community Hospitals.* Oxfordshire Health Authority/ Distance Learning Centre

Liddiard P 1989 Personal communication

Open University 1984 *A Systematic Approach to Nursing Care.* The Open University Press

Open University 1988 *Professional Judgment.* The Open University Press.

Rafferty A M and Robinson K S M 1988 *The Nursing Workforce.* Distance Learning Centre

Robinson K S M and Vaughan B 1988 *Images of Nursing.* Distance Learning Centre

Schon D A 1983 *Reflective Practitioner.* M T Smith

SCROLL 1987 *Thinking About Social Care.* Cranfield Press

Vaughan B 1989 Two roles one job, *Nursing Times* 85 *11* p52

7 The role of the open learning editor

Jan Fordham

The development of printed open learning materials for the nursing profession presents a special challenge for the editor. In part, this derives from the nature of open learning itself which demands the generation of materials that differ significantly from conventional textbooks. In part, however, the challenge arises from the way in which the role of the editor is perceived, both in the world of education in which open learning is largely rooted and in that of nursing which provides its context and content. Unlikely to be a nurse, the editor is sometimes seen as being somewhat peripheral to the 'real' business of developing materials. This chapter seeks to argue, however, that the editor occupies a central role in the developmental and production process, a role which is becoming increasingly diverse and valued and which demands an array of specialist skills.

In 1983, writing about open learning in an international context, Jenkins argued that:

> Course writers demand training. Gone are the days when the novice writer would confidently set about the task of writing with only minimal guidance. Gone are the days of experiment, when the enthusiastic writer would, unaided, become aware of the problems of teaching by correspondence and creatively adapt his or her classroom techniques to teaching at a distance. Gone are the days when the intervention of an editor or educational technologist was considered a wrongful intrusion into the preserve of a teacher!

Experience suggests that this is not necessarily true in the field of nursing. Now that open learning is becoming more widely accepted, it is sometimes seen largely as a cheap and convenient substitute for conventional face-to-face-teaching. As a result, it is not uncommon to find individual nurse educators, or small groups, embarking on the development of an open learning package under the impression that it need involve little more than a reworking of their lecture notes. The skills and resources required to develop practice-based materials that are educationally sound and intellectually challenging, and that stimulate and motivate learners, are often sadly underestimated.

The reality is that the production of high quality learning materials relies on a foundation of extensive experience or specific training. The implications of this are that, in the context of open learning, nurse educators must either speedily acquire skills which they have probably never needed before or learn to share part of their traditional domain without feeling threatened by a sense of encroachment of boundaries. In conventional educational settings, teachers exercise almost complete control over the process of teaching; although working within the framework of a curriculum and requiring some administrative and technical support, the teacher establishes a direct relationship with students and operates relatively independently within the classroom. As Thorpe (1988) suggests, however, open learning does not necessarily diminish the role of this key figure, but it does change it – and it also increases the importance of other staff roles. Not only can the open learning teacher not talk directly to those she is teaching, she is unlikely to be able to negotiate the various components of the publishing process which enables her to make contact with them. In developing open learning materials, then, the teacher cannot be independent of others.

From manuscript to print

The production of printed matter has been described by Rogers (1985) as a kind of 'creative conveyor belt'. Ideas plus materials plus labour are loaded on at one end and completed publications are offloaded at the other.' For most of us, books are such an integral part of our lives that we tend to give little more than a passing thought to anything but the content of the final product; nor should we, since the art of publishing is to present the author's work in an attractive, stimulating and satisfying form which facilitates communication between writer and reader. Nevertheless, the publication process obviously needs more than an author and requires the input of a team of specialists, largely invisible to the consumer, with defined roles and expertise that are called into play at specific points in the developmental cycle. In the preparation of open learning materials, this process is often structured in such a way that there is a clear separation between academic and production functions, with the editor generally being seen as belonging to the production arena, together with the typist or word processor operator, the designer, the production manager, the typesetter and the printer. What is sometimes forgotten, however, is that it is the editor who cements the link between nursing, education and publishing in order to transform an author's manuscript into an accessible and effective tool for professional development; as such, she requires experience and skills drawn from all three worlds.

Rogers (1985) defines the editor as 'the guardian of a book's style, content and logic'; in the context of open learning, the editor is also the ultimate custodian of the quality of the interaction between teacher and learner in the materials which are designed as the major focus of a course of study. Like a juggler, she must keep her eye on several balls at the same time: on the content and purpose of what the author is saying, and whether this is being communicated effectively to the learner; on the objectives of the programme as a whole, and whether the publication is consistent in style, presentation and quality with other materials in a series; and, most importantly, on the learner, and whether the materials facilitate a process both of active learning and of personal and professional development. A meticulous and, indeed, fastidious eye for detail thus needs to be combined with a sound understanding of educational principles and key issues in nursing, an intelligent approach to content and an empathetic understanding of what it can feel like to be a learner who is geographically separated from the teacher.

The open learning teacher

For the editor, into whose hands the final manuscript is passed, the demands of the task ahead depend considerably on the open learning and writing skills of the author. When a teacher is an experienced writer who can produce text which is well-constructed, fluent and imaginative and who keeps the needs of the learner firmly in mind, the editor's role is relatively straightforward. When a teacher is relatively new to open learning or is unused to writing, however, a greater input is required of the editor.

Whilst open learning has been well established in the UK for more than two decades, its acceptance within nursing has been much more recent. By their very nature, the majority of open learning materials for nurses need to be prepared by nurses with specialist areas of nursing knowledge; the wide range of materials now required to complement conventional pre- and post-registration education demands that even projects specifically established to develop open learning programmes for nurses, such as the Distance Learning Centre at South Bank Polytechnic and Continuing Nurse Education at Barnet College, have to commission external authors to develop materials. The pool of nurse educators with expertise in open learning is, however, still comparatively small; developing high quality open learning material is an art in itself and subject specialists who are excellent face-to-face communicators do not necessarily write easily or well. Even experienced writers often find difficulty in coping with the informal style and interactive approach required in an open learning package and it is not uncommon to find that materials are more subject-oriented than learner-oriented. Special skills are, after all, required to interest, inform and maintain the motivation of learners with a wide range of professional concerns and experience, and different levels of academic ability, with whom the teacher is unlikely ever to have any personal contact.

From copy editor to transformer

The transformation of good content into good open learning material may thus demand the involvement of educational technologists who do not necessarily have – or need – in-depth knowledge of the subject matter, but who do have experience of open learning. In this respect, open and distance learning may offer some advantages over classroom-based study where a translator is, sometimes wrongly, considered unnecessary. Rowntree (1986) defines such a person as a 'transformer: a skilled communicator who can liaise with any subject specialists whose writing is obscure, winkling out their key ideas and re-expressing them in ways the learners will be able to understand.' This person is sometimes a core academic member of the team although the editor, who normally works more closely with the text than anyone except the author, is also a logical occupant of this role. Nevertheless, in educational or professional institutions where the majority of open learning projects are based, the role of the editor is often seen as being largely confined to copy-editing, a process which begins only when the completed manuscript is handed over by the author for production and which involves the polishing of the text – ensuring that spelling and grammatical errors are corrected, that there are no inconsistencies in style or format and that the text flows easily – and the preparation of the manuscript for typesetting and printing. This is an essential function that is all too often undervalued; however, the educational and creative aspects of the open learning editor's role – the equivalent to what, in conventional publishing, is termed 'sub-editing' or developmental editing – are also frequently underestimated.

A continuum of roles can thus be contained by the title 'editor' although the extent to which materials require the input of a transformer rather than simply that of a copy editor largely depends on the quality of individual authors' manuscripts. While this spectrum of functions can be performed by the same person, this may not be an effective use of an experienced editor's skills since a higher level of expertise and familiarity with educational and nursing issues is required for the transformer role; a small project with limited staff resources may, however, have no alternative. It is important to recognise, though, that just as an experienced nurse educator doesn't necessarily make a good writer of open learning materials, an experienced editor doesn't necessarily make a good open learning editor or a good transformer; open learning requires increased numbers of specialist staff who can offer a combination of these educational and technical skills. Foremost amongst these are an understanding of the nature of effective open learning materials and the needs and characteristics of the end-user.

'Why can't a unit be more like a book?'

A key element of the open learning editor's role is developing a partnership with authors, some of whom encounter real difficulties in making the transition from writing lecture notes, course handouts, journal articles or books to writing open learning materials. The new open learning author's predicament is well illustrated by a letter to *Teaching at a Distance*; writing in 1981, Jeffcoate described how, although having considerable experience of writing, an activity which he found enjoyable, preparing Open University materials was 'more of a struggle and less of a pleasure, and the end product none the better for either' because of the kind of writing that is expected of unit authors. Having posed the question 'Why can't a unit be more like a book?' he suggests:

> The answer, I imagine, would be that a unit is a *teaching* text and must therefore include something called *pedagogy*. In this context, pedagogy seems to mean two things: engaging students in a kind of avuncular chat to soften them up and then subjecting them to the hoops and hurdles of questions and activities. I have to say, I find the first ploy patronizing, if not insulting; as to the second, I cannot understand how activities survive. My experience from summer school is that students ignore them, and with good reason. So would I... Need a unit do more than meet the [following] conditions?... that it should be lucid, readable and entertaining; that it should be candid about its intentions, assumptions and limitations; and, if arguing a case, that it should make plain the nature of the evidence the case rests on. What else could students, pressed for time, possibly want? Has anyone asked them? As for the mythology of the 'interactive text', any text is that. How successfully interactive a text is depends on how well written it is, not on how many activities it includes.

Open learning materials for nurses are designed as professional development tools rather than as academic texts, and learners are therefore likely to want more than Jeffcoate was, at least in 1981, apparently willing to acknowledge. A reply to his letter by Iley (1983) provides a succinct answer to his question:

> Reading a book is not the same as studying it and the major
> reason we write units and not books is that we are attempting to
> teach students the skills of handling information as well as the
> information itself... it is better to attempt to teach how skills can
> be used appropriately and with purpose than to hope that,
> somehow, students will develop them.

Interactivity

It is interactivity, a hallmark of good open learning materials, that
creates opportunities for learners to practise these skills and
encourages them to relate the information, issues and ideas contained
in the text to their own needs and experiences; as Paley (1985)
expresses it, 'the material provides a screen on to which the learner
can project herself'. Interactive open learning material thus combines
the information-giving role of the textbook with the guidance,
motivation and support role of the classroom teacher who provides
practice and feedback. For Holmberg (1986):

> The communication element is rightly considered a corner stone
> of distance education; the more it resembles conversations –
> naturally premeditated and well-prepared – the better... when
> real didactic conversation cannot take place it is the spirit and
> atmosphere of conversation that should – and largely do –
> characterize distance education.

This process involves both simulated and real conversation: a
conversation-like interaction between the writer-tutor and the learner
through the medium of the course materials, and real conversation
between the learner and the tutor-counsellor or facilitator through
written, face-to-face or telephone interaction. To be effective, this
conversation must be structured from the perspective of the learner,
rather than that of the teacher; subject experts cannot know the extent
of their students' expertise but they must seek to engage them in active
dialogue which fully acknowledges their contribution to the
conversation as being both valid and valuable.

Moreover, while all good open learning materials require the potential
for active connections to be made between the ideas of the teacher
and the learner, vocationally-oriented open learning materials for
nurses demand a process of tripartite interaction in which the
dimension of practice has a prominent place. Thus, interactive devices
such as in-text questions, activities and exercises are often designed to
guide students out of the materials, as well as through them, and into

an exploration of their own attitudes, skills and practical experience, both personal and professional. Indeed, in their *Interim Report on an Evaluation of the Use of Distance Learning Materials for Continuing Professional Education for Nurses, Midwives and Health Visitors*, Lawrence, Maggs and Rogers (1988) report that a key reason cited by respondents for the use of open and distance learning materials is this learner-centred approach which enables learners to link theoretical and conceptual issues with their work experiences. Consider the example shown in Figures 7.1 and 7.2 taken from the Distance Learning Centre study pack *Improving Teamwork* (Isard, 1987) which, in considering what management is, encourages learners to reflect on the managerial elements of their own roles and responsibilities.

Consider another example (Figure 7.3), this time from the Open University course, *Caring for Older People*.

In her research on alternative uses of materials produced by the Health and Social Welfare section of the Open University's Centre for Continuing Education, Stainton Rogers (1984) found that activities of this kind could have a profound influence on attitudes. She cites the student who commented on this activity:

> The topic about giving up your home and going into an EPH, I see that in a different light now. I can see what a big upheaval that can be and how much it could affect their lives... because I've thought about it myself, if I was going to give up my home – what would I take that was precious to me? There's so many things you'd want to keep.

Often, however, the demands of interactivity cause difficulty for the inexperienced writer of open learning materials and it is here that the most creative elements of the editor's role come into play. The drafts prepared by some writers suggest a sense of discomfort at moving away from a subject-centred approach to one which is learner-centred and it is not uncommon to find texts which hint that activities have been added on, rather than being designed as an integral part of the work. For the editor, then, the challenge lies in joining the seams, ensuring that the text flows smoothly into and out of activities and exercises. She must also be alert to further opportunities for interaction, suggesting activities that reinforce the text, promote conceptual links with personal experience and facilitate retention. Clearly, every activity must have a purpose; what is equally important, however, is that this should be obvious and relevant to the learner. It is the editor's responsibility to ensure that the activity is constructed in such a way that learners are conscious of how it will contribute to their development by guiding them through a process of testing and

Motivator ——→

Guidance
on
completing
activity ——→

Activity
cues ←——

Feedback ←——

Recognition
of learner's
experience ←——

Personal
example
from
author ←——

Managing scarce resources

You may feel that you are only in charge of your work area for limited periods of time – for example, as a staff nurse in charge while the sister is away. That alone would say a great deal about how you view yourself in relation to others in the team, particularly the person you deem to be the leader. Nevertheless, if this is how you feel at the moment, then try to see your work on this study pack both as being directly relevant for you during the specific times when you are in charge and as a preparation for when you later take on this responsibility on a formal basis.

In the next activity we want you to find out what resources you are responsible for during the course of a day. First, however, let's look at the main categories in more detail.

Space

- approximately how much space, in square feet/yards does your work area cover? (this space costs money in terms of repairs, electricity, water, heating and lighting)
- in the community, how many square miles do you cover? How many households come within your caseload? What is your average daily mileage?

Staff

- how many staff are there available in your work area and what are their grades?
- what are the cost implications of these staff – both directly to the organisation as a whole and indirectly? For instance, what are their future training needs?
- how are these training needs and planned experiences to be met, particularly in times of diminishing resources?

Consumable items

- what items do you and your staff use over the course of a day? For instance, C.S.S.D., dressings, laundry, stationery, petrol. If you have a sympathetic stores manager you may be able to work out the exact cost.

Now turn on Activity 1.3

You have now outlined what you are responsible *for*, that is, the location and resources you have at your disposal. Now it is time to explore what you *do* as a manager. Think back over the last day or two at work and jot down the *actions* you have performed that you could classify as 'management'.

Now turn to Activity 1.4

One of the problems you may have encountered when making up your list is that there may have been some overlap between nursing tasks and nursing management and that it was difficult, therefore, to identify what was purely management.

'NURSING' AND 'MANAGING'

The role of the nurse as a manager can be difficult to define and you perhaps found when you first qualified that changing from being a student to being 'in charge' was very stressful, partly because you were not absolutely sure of what your role was, let alone how to do it. One reason for this could be that, for students, nurses performing 'real nursing' have high prestige.

Personal example

When I became a ward sister I was distressed at how rarely I was able to perform direct care, except at weekends or other quiet times. I would have enjoyed doing this, and was conscious that my staff would view my lack of 'hands on' real work with disapproval. However, I was always being interrupted whenever I attempted to do 'real' nursing. The telephone would ring and it would be a problem that senior students could not manage; a visitor would arrive on the ward wanting to see me; a problem would arise.

Figure 7.1   Interactivity: reflecting on managerial elements of learner's own role

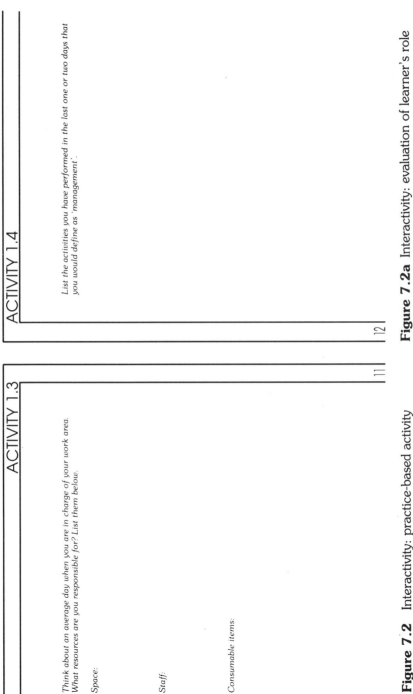

ACTIVITY 1.4

List the activities you have performed in the last one or two days that you would define as 'management'.

12

Figure 7.2a Interactivity: evaluation of learner's role

ACTIVITY 1.3

Think about an average day when you are in charge of your work area. What resources are you responsible for? List them below.

Space:

Staff:

Consumable items:

11

Figure 7.2 Interactivity: practice-based activity

increasing their skills, and building new ones. If this is not apparent, students may well see the interactive elements of the text as 'the hoops and hurdles of questions and activities' described by Jeffcoate.

Activity 11.4

Choosing what to take

You are being admitted to the local old people's home, where you will be fortunate enough to have a room of your own but it is fully furnished. It has a small modern dressing-table with three drawers, a wardrobe which is 2'6" long, a bedside locker and a window ledge 5' long and 6" wide. No belongings, including clothes, can be stored elsewhere, or in cases. Decide what you will take: the space is roughly the equivalent of what can be packed in a 'largish' suitcase.

Figure 7.3   Interactivity: encouraging learners to relate to their own needs and experiences

Style and tone

Activities and exercises are by no means the only interactive components of open learning material. Indeed, the overall style and tone of the text as a whole should seek to create something of the flavour of a face-to-face session. Where the learner has no direct contact with the writer-tutor, however, the modulation of the voice and the non-verbal gestures and cues that are an essential part of the communication process somehow have to be conveyed through the medium of a flat page. Every open learning producer appreciates feedback from students who say that they can almost hear the tutor speaking to them as they work through the materials. The skill, then, is in writing materials that sustain the characteristics of didactic conversation whilst meeting rigorous academic and professional standards.

Some writers appear to be uncomfortable about moving away from the style that is appropriate for the professional journal or book, seeming to fear that using a direct form of address, posing questions – and sometimes replies – and using simple language undermines a text's academic credibility and insults the student. Elgood (1987) suggests that ' ... those who create distance learning material will probably have their roots in the educational world and may, unknowingly, have beliefs about what may or may not be done, and what is or is not respectable, that limit their options and are not really appropriate to the work in hand.' As Race (1987) comments, however, 'The only people who tend to be insulted by simple language in learning material seem to be academics! I believe this is evidence of elitism in our ranks!'

'User-friendly' is a term commonly used in the open learning world to describe an approach which demonstrates that the writer-tutor is on the learner's side and will do everything possible to facilitate learning;

the choice of language which aids comprehension and stimulates enjoyment is an essential element of this approach. Simple language does not automatically mean simple concepts, although in trying to address the interests and needs of a disparate group of students with a common interest, there is a danger of writing for the lowest common denominator; in trying to avoid the trap of preparing materials which are too formal or academic in their approach and adopting a style which is friendly and informal, it is all too easy to go too far the other way and come across as being casual, unprofessional or patronising. It is the editor's job, therefore, to ensure that the materials are pitched at a level which is both accessible and acceptable to learners, from the practitioner with five O-levels to the graduate nurse.

Understanding the end-user

It is, in fact, the diversity of the student population that provides the major challenge for the editor of open learning materials since the end-users must, of course, be the focus of all our work. Although united by an interest in a particular subject, they have a wide range of educational experiences, learning abilities and professional expertise and have differing motivations and expectations of their study. If the concept of 'user-friendliness' is to have any real meaning, it must be manifested through a recognition of what it feels like to be a learner, perhaps working at home after a tiring and stressful day with learning materials spread out over the dining-room table after the children have gone to bed or studying during quiet periods on the ward at night. Nurses studying open learning materials spend most of their study time alone; the open learning producer has a responsibility to strive to ensure that they do not feel isolated.

Open learning may, nevertheless, sometimes seem a lonely path to follow which is why the support of a tutor-counsellor and contact with fellow learners in group sessions is an important complement to individual work on study packs. The interactive nature of good materials does mean, however, that the open learner cannot take refuge at the back of the classroom or rely on her peers' opinions to shape her own. Not only is she being presented with new concepts; more importantly, she is urged to question her own ideas and beliefs, a process which may be uncomfortable and even threatening if it results in a recognition of the need for change. The open learning student undertaking a course in literature may find an exploration of the development of the twentieth century novel to be intellectually stimulating and emotionally enriching. The nurse who becomes an open learner, however, is confronted with a much more direct and personal challenge which demands an active and individual response. Not only is she encouraged to reflect on what she has been taught and what she has learned from her own experience, she is asked to critically evaluate her own, and her colleagues', practice and to determine what action may be required. The implications of this are by no means always welcome. While it may be easier to think through difficult issues in peace and quiet rather than in the work environment or the classroom, the open learning student grappling with concepts or activities with which she may feel uncomfortable needs a sense of security about the quality of the materials which are asking her to engage in this challenging process and to know that *her* needs are recognised as being paramount. The editor has the ultimate responsibility to serve as the learner's advocate, filtering the materials through a fine mesh of realism and even scepticism, and eliminating as many barriers to effective learning as possible, whilst ensuring that the learner is still intellectually challenged and stretched.

For many nurses, educated in a system where questioning is often discouraged, it is not easy to become an independent learner who critically evaluates and actively uses information rather than simply absorbing it. At some level, many of us subconsciously hold the belief that if something is published in a book it must be correct. Somehow the printed page conveys an authority that encourages us to suspend critical awareness and that legitimises the content, even if that content is unambiguously an author's personal opinion: 'It must be right, otherwise they wouldn't have published it'. The corollary to this is often 'If I don't understand it, it's my fault because I'm not intelligent enough', a powerful dampener of motivation. Jeffcoate (1981), however, again provides an example of how some academics find it difficult to relinquish an teacher-centred rather than learner-centred approach:

> We seem to have reached the point where there is actually too much commenting, too much drafting, too much editing, too much general interference with the unit author's rights – and certainly far too long a gestation period between the original conception and the eventual birth. The net result is that, in the interests of excluding anything which might be construed as polemical, tendentious or flamboyant, academic nervousness and stylistic anonymity prevail. Obviously there is a danger of students being bamboozled by ideology and intimidated by a hectoring style, but I would have thought that, provided the conditions for a good unit I have listed were fulfilled, students were old enough to look after themselves.

Are learners able to look after themselves, though? It certainly cannot be assumed that this is the case. At the risk of being seen to interfere with the rights of the author, the editor has to assert that learners have rights too; if their needs are ultimately to have priority, as they should, this may necessitate substantial rewriting of the materials, wherever possible in consultation with the author. The editor knows that some authors simply do not write well or know how to prepare materials for a non-academic audience and, indeed, few have been trained to do so; whilst some readily acknowledge that their expertise lies in the domain of content rather than writing technique, the editor certainly requires an array of interpersonal skills to smooth ruffled feelings and foster a harmonious partnership with an author that promotes a fusion of their complementary skills.

A key task for the editor may thus involve interpreting the material for the learner since the specialist knowledge that is essential for the development of the materials sometimes serves to mask the meaning. Nursing is such a heterogeneous profession that nurse specialists sometimes forget what non-specialists don't know; the subject-matter may be so familiar to authors or the objectives underlying activities so obvious that they fail to recognise why they may be a source of bewilderment or anxiety to learners. However, *Ensuring Quality in Open Learning: A handbook for action* (Manpower Services Commission, 1988), a code of practice for open learning producers and deliverers, specifically states that producers should make their materials totally self-explanatory 'so that, at any point within them, Learners always understand what they are supposed to be doing, and how and why they should be doing it.'

In the classroom, the learner who doesn't understand something can ask a question; the open learning approach, by its very nature, means that the author and learner are separated. A learner who is bogged down by ambiguity, inconsistency or apparent irrelevance, none of which are unknown in authors' manuscripts, is at risk of developing a sense of inadequacy or desperation, and this must be avoided at all costs. The editor must therefore carefully assess whether the text says what the author means and whether it says it in a way which the learner will find accessible and comprehensible. Inconsistencies in the use of terminology or concepts that are a particular danger when a number of contributors tackle the same subject must be ironed out; jargon must be defined, new concepts explained and their relevance made clear. Armed with the motto 'Never completely trust an author' and with the image of 'the unknown learner' firmly in mind, she must constantly seek to check and clarify, all the time using those essential questions in the editorial vocabulary: 'why?', 'how?' and 'how is this point relevant?' This does not mean that she seeks to remove all the features of a text that encourage learners to make the conceptual leaps that are a vital and satisfying part of learning. What it does mean, however, is that she ensures that the stepping stones are adequately signposted and not too far apart. After all, negative emotions such as boredom, confusion and anxiety tend to focus attention on the source of distress and serve to block off all forms of effective learning. Nevertheless, Snell (1987) reminds us that:

...where the intention is to provide learners with the opportunity for development, it is very likely that they will experience a measure of emotional pain or discomfort resulting from both the new insight they may gain into themselves and the very process of moving from the known and familiar into the unknown. To seek to prevent such pain in such circumstances is tantamount to attempting to block personal development, as the risk of some pain seems to be inherent in learning of this nature, rather like the growing pains some children experience.

In some respects, this pain can be likened to that sometimes felt during physical exercise. A nurse pursuing an open learning programme may know it's going to do her good, but if the experience is too uncomfortable and ultimately not enjoyable, motivation will flag and good intentions fall by the wayside.

Format and presentation

While this process of self-examination and personal growth is an integral part of effective learning, the producers of open learning materials can anticipate some of the potential sources of pain and discomfort. One means of achieving this is to maximise the 'open' nature of the materials. 'Openness' implies that as many barriers to learning are removed as possible and that learners – and not only teachers – have control over learning. One of the obvious benefits of open and distance learning is, of course, that learners can be freed from the confines of a study timetable which may not fit easily with personal or work commitments and can thus make decisions for themselves about the time, place and pace of their study.

The concept of 'openness' goes beyond this, however; to some degree, the extent to which materials are 'open' is reflected in the way in which they are designed. The structuring of a course or study pack so that modules or chapters are largely self-contained, for example, offers learners choice about whether they wish to follow a linear approach or to tackle topics in an order that meets their own immediate needs and interests. The division of the material into sections that require two or three hours of study offers them both manageable goals for individual study sessions and obvious stopping places, thus assisting them to plan how they might use their study time most effectively. A well-designed structure, with an informative introduction, chapter titles and sub-headings can help them to see where they are going in a study pack and where they can take short cuts, skimming through certain sections or skipping ones which cover familiar ground. The inclusion of aims at the beginning of a study pack or chapter can also help them to decide what they feel will be of use to them and what they wish to study; conversely, presented in the form of 'Now you have completed this chapter, you should be able to... ' they provide learners with an opportunity to decide for themselves whether they have understood the key concepts and whether further consolidation is needed before they move on to another topic.

Where formal assessment procedures are built into an open learning programme, as with the Distance Learning Centre's Diploma in Nursing, feedback cannot be immediate since assignments must pass through a rigorous process of assessment. Learners can be encouraged to assess their own work, however; self-assessment questions offer them a further means of checking their understanding through comparing their answers with those of the author and thus of gauging their own progress. Similarly, activities which ask them to engage in a process of reflection, or to carry out an exercise or practical task and subsequently evaluate their achievement, provide developmental markers which both help to keep motivation levels up and to highlight areas where tutorial support may be needed. Activities which invite learners to involve their colleagues, through joint problem-solving exercises, for example, enable them to share and discuss their new knowledge and insights with the team in which they work and open up opportunities for peer assessment and support. Such devices all offer means of extending the degree of control which learners have over their own study and shifting the emphasis from the passive receipt of information to active involvement in learning.

Materials which have a clear and attractive design that consciously seeks to avoid reawakening memories of school textbooks and homework can help to convey the notion that learning can be stimulating and enjoyable. Headings, illustrations and cartoons can be used to break up solid blocks of text that might otherwise look intimidating or dull. Wide margins inviting learners to add their comments or blank spaces encouraging them to write down their responses to activities enable them to construct an individualised learning tool that draws together the author's insights with their own in Holmberg's process of didactic conversation. An effective interface between the author, editor and designer is thus essential in creating a format that reflects the purpose and integrity of the materials and which welcomes the learner to interact with them.

New technology

The issues that we have considered here indicate that a considerable input is required for the production of printed open learning materials after the author has gratefully added the last full stop to the manuscript. Until comparatively recently, this process was to some extent constrained by the technology available: the laborious typing and retyping of drafts and edited manuscripts often subconsciously

E

served as a check on what was perceived to be feasible in the time available before material was passed on to the typesetter. The advent of word-processing and desk-top publishing has opened up new possibilities in the development of high quality materials, offering a far greater element of control than ever before over the production and reproduction process. Text, graphics and layout can be finalised on computer disc which can then be sent for computerised typesetting, thus enabling the galley proof and page proof stage to be bypassed before printing. Alternatively, the laser printer enables cost-effective and attractively-presented materials to be produced using photocopying for small numbers of learners where printing is not economically viable.

Timmers (1986), cited in Rumble (1986), describes the effects of introducing computer-based technology on the development of the second half of a chemistry course at the Open Learning Institute in British Columbia, Canada. When all members of the course team were provided with a microcomputer and training materials on how to use it, the nature of authoring changed; the assessor knew that the author could easily revise the text so the comments were more extensive, editing was easier because the text was 'cleaner' and queries and amendments could be inserted into the text, and the writer was more involved in discussing and agreeing editorial changes. Particularly significant was the result that the time needed to produce completed pages for printing dropped from 120 to 50 hours per page, with subsequent financial savings. The development of new technology has thus substantially increased the cost-effectiveness and flexibility of the production process.

Who makes a good open learning editor?

The increasing use of computer-based technology in publishing means, however, that the open learning editor has had to add yet another area of expertise to her repertoire. Not until the mid-1980s did open learning find a place for itself in nursing; with rapidly increasing recognition of its benefits, particularly in the light of the implications of Project 2000 for nurse education, its role is constantly expanding. The role of the open learning editor is similarly growing. She must keep abreast of changes within the nursing profession as well as in the world of open learning, of new developments in education as well as in publishing.

What kind of person makes a good open learning editor? Even with years of publishing experience, an editor who knows little about nursing will find it difficult to spot inaccuracies in the text or make a useful contribution to the content. One who is herself a nurse, or is familiar with nursing, but who has limited knowledge of the principles of adult education or open learning may lack the educational dimension that is crucial to an understanding of what helps learners to learn most effectively. An experienced educator without extensive copy-editing and sub-editing skills and an eye for design will have to learn a range of technical skills in order to be able to ensure the quality of presentation that should be a hallmark of all open learning materials for nurses.

A new breed of editor is now emerging. In my own case, the route into this diverse role was through training and experience in health education and community development, the commissioning and writing of educational materials and, only latterly, editing. Having entered the world of open learning when it first reached out into nursing, much of my expertise has developed from a blend of knowledge and practical experience gained in a variety of professional contexts rather than from formal training. There are, of course, many other possible entry points.

As open learning expands further in nursing, what is now vital is a recognition of the need for increasing numbers of specialist open learning editors – or educational technologists or 'transformers': a new term will probably have to be found to reflect the unique nature of this function. While the accompanying need for training may pose problems for small projects which are new to publishing or open learning, open learning itself can offer practical assistance; the National Extension College study pack, *Editing for Everyone* (Hall, 1983), for example, offers a useful grounding in basic copy-editing and proof-reading skills. Texts such as *Teaching through Self-instruction: A practical handbook for course developers* (Rowntree, 1986) provide guidance on the development and production of materials. Nevertheless, an open learning nursing editor is not born overnight. Nurse educators must be prepared to invest time and resources into the development of new skills – or to welcome and value new people with skills that complement their own.

References

Elgood C 1987 Motivating learners, in Hodgson, V E, Mann, S J and Snell, R (eds), *Beyond Distance Teaching – Towards Open Learning*, The Society for Research into Higher Education & Open University Press.

Hall C 1983 *Editing for Everyone*, National Extension College.

Holmberg B 1986 *Growth and Structure of Distance Education*, Croom Helm.

Iley J 1983 Why a unit is not a book, *Teaching at a Distance*, 23, Summer pp76-77.

Isard J 1987 *Improving Teamwork*, Distance Learning Centre.

Jeffcoate R 1981 Why can't a unit be more like a book?, *Teaching at a Distance*, 20, Winter, pp776.

Jenkins J 1983 Tell me how to write, in Sewart D, Keegan D and Holmberg B (eds), *Distance Education: International perspectives*, Croom Helm.

Lawrence J, Maggs C and Rogers J 1988 *Interim Report on an Evaluation of the Use of Distance Learning Materials for Continuing Professional Education for Nurses, Midwives and Health Visitors*, Institute of Education, University of London.

Manpower Services Commission 1988 *Ensuring Quality in Open Learning: A handbook for action*, MSC.

Paley J 1985 *Open Learning and the Caring Professions: Some concepts and implications*, unpublished paper, Cranfield Institute of Technology.

Race P 1987 *Tone and Style for Open Learning*, The Scottish Central Institutions Committee for Educational Development.

Rogers G 1985 *Editing for Print*, Macdonald.

Rowntree D 1986 *Teaching through Self-instruction: A practical handbook for course developers*, Kogan Page.

Rumble G 1986 *The Planning and Management of Distance Education*, Croom Helm.

Snell R 1987 The challenge of painful and unpleasant emotions, in Hodgson V E, Mann S J and Snell R (eds), *Beyond Distance Teaching – Towards open learning*, The Society for Research into Higher Education & Open University Press.

Spencer D C 1980 *Thinking About Open Learning Systems*, Council for Educational Technology.

Stainton Rogers W 1984 Alternative uses of materials: research findings, *Teaching at a Distance*, 25, Autumn, pp58-68.

Thorpe M 1988) *Evaluating Open and Distance Learning*, Longman.

Timmers S 1986 Microcomputers in course development, *Programmed Learning and Educational Technology*, 23 (1), pp123.

8 Choosing and using media

Fiona Munro

The fact that something is possible doesn't necessarily make it desirable, and the purpose of this chapter is to explore both what is available in terms of educational technology and what the potential use might be of each of these technologies (media) in nurse education. One danger in using new technologies is that the range of technical possibilities can displace other considerations, such as educational goals, the learning environment and the organisational environment of the educational institution. So we need to start by re-emphasising three fundamental questions which have to be answered when considering any teaching medium:

- who are we teaching
- where are they learning
- what are they learning?

The focus here will be on the impact of technology on these issues; not so much what the technologies do in the abstract, as what they can do for you and for your learners.

Some problems and principles

The role of the educational technologist is to stand back from the content of teaching a particular subject and examine the art form itself. As far as open learning and the use of media is concerned, the literature and research tends towards examining either the role of mass media in education or the role of media in mass education. Little has yet been done in terms of model-building for the small-scale or local-initiative type of resource-based educational enterprise. Although this doesn't necessarily detract from the usefulness of available models, it does need to be borne in mind. The educational media models themselves tackle three major issues:

- instructional design
- cost and resource analysis
- comparison of 'intrinsic' features of each medium.

However, approaches to adult education have been changing rapidly during this decade, with an increased emphasis on the role of the learner, so models for instructional design and media selection based on traditional teaching paradigms need to be treated with caution. As Duchastel argues:

> Traditional Instructional Design (ID) is strongly centred on the clear specification of learning objectives and the design of instructional interventions geared to these objectives. It involves a style of design which created learning environments that are directive, ie in which the learner is led towards the mastery of the learning objectives through specified procedures...
>
> Duchastel 1988

Duchastel argues for a more learner centred approach and the '...need to explore a wider design model for instructional products...' by creating a responsive learning environment which allows learners to adopt an inquiry approach to learning. Further, Knowles (1984) commends the concept of andragogy, which proposes that adult learners should participate in decisions about the teaching and learning process, with the emphasis on collaboration and support. Such new ideas, all sharing in common a learner centred approach abound. Together with what is already known about individual differences in the quality of learning from educational media, the implication is that students should have the opportunity to select their learning of any given subject from a range of media, in order to maximise effective learning. This casts new light on media selection models which propose taxonomies of the type of learning best facilitated by each medium, and shifts the whole debate towards individual learning styles rather than 'best' delivery media. The utility of any media selection model therefore rests in the context of a well developed plan for delivering open learning to a specific group of learners.

The physical characteristics of media

One of the difficulties in evaluating any medium is trying to discover what is actually involved in producing learning materials in that medium. Educational technologists have a tendency to presuppose a familiarity with the physical characteristics if each medium amongst their readers which renders unnecessary any explanation beyond a discussion of their educational characteristics. If you are amongst the vast majority who don't possess this knowledge, the following brief explanations might help to fill in any gaps.

Print

Without wishing to state the obvious, there are a number of ways of using print-based technology in an educational setting. Existing textbooks are used as a learning resource in nearly all educational environments, but constructing open learning courseware will demand the generation of print-based materials of some kind, and needs to be thought about in the same context as other media.

In terms of the generation of printed material which will eventually end up on the learners' lap, two processes are involved; one is the generation of the 'master copy' of the material and the other involves its reproduction. Different forms of reproduction demand different levels of perfection of the master, and the economics of reproduction means that decisions have to be made about reproduction well before the master is originated. Reproduction quality decisions are a product of the nature of the contents (eg whether or not photographs, colour plates, illustrations, etc. are to be incorporated with the text), the volume to be reproduced, and the size of the budget.

Originating the master using traditional publishing methods might well cost three times as much as the printing costs. The origination costs include typing or word-processing the text, commissioning or buying photographs and having them prepared for print, commissioning text design and other artwork, professional editing, keyed typesetting, and paste-up for camera ready copy. Most publishers allow a timescale of between six and nine months for the origination process alone. Using new technology can bypass some of the iterative processes of origination and can reduce the costs and timescales involved in typesetting and editing but, of itself, does not have any impact on conventional print costs. Using personal microcomputers to generate text and using this as input for electronic typesetting reduces both time and cost. Going further, using desktop publishing (DTP) systems (eg Ventura, Pagemaker) can reduce the costs of generating integrated text, graphics and paste-up and can also be used to generate typeset pages by sending the data in disk form (or down the telephone line) to a typesetter. While DTP can also be used directly to generate a master (which saves on phototypesetting costs), only the new generation of laser printers produces a sufficiently dense image for successful conventional print reproduction, although laser prints are usually more than adequate for photocopied reproduction.

Photocopying facilities range from the crude to the sophisticated, and the producer needs to know the limitations of the equipment that will be used before making decisions about the physical content and make-up of the master. Generally speaking, photocopying is slower than conventional printing, the quality of reproduction is poorer than print, and it can cost the same or more over a certain 'run size' (reproduction volume). Despite this, photocopying has often been used successfully to produce attractive materials. Although there is an obvious attraction of DTP for the producer since it means that there is control over the material at all stages, the other side of that coin is the danger of getting sucked into the physical process of origination at the expense of academic and educational considerations.

Audio

Professional voice recording is still based on tape technology, where the voice signal is picked up by a microphone and fed through a mixer which can be used to enhance the signal and recorded on magnetic tape on a multichannel reel-to-reel machine at a speed which will allow for ease of editing. Advances in technology have meant that this signal can now be digitised and manipulated electronically, and this technique is largely used for music recordings. The editing process involves cutting and splicing the tape to remove unwanted material, to add material from another source, to make the material fit a specified time frame, or to change the presentation order of the material. The edited tape constitutes the master version which is used for subsequent reproduction. There are two methods of reproduction onto audio cassette: the 'bin' method which involves making a secondary master but provides a high quality of multiple copying at high speed, or the dubbing method which involves creating a master cassette and equipment which will dub a number of cassettes simultaneously. A major problem in originating the master is that the end result must be very 'clean', with a satisfactory signal-to-noise ratio, because the act of reproducing tape introduces more ambient noise and the voice signal deteriorates accordingly. Compact disc technology overcomes this problem by digitilising the signal and storing it in the way described later in this chapter for videodisc. Although it can produce 'perfect' results, compact disc technology is very expensive both in origination and reproduction relative to tape technology. Audio cassettes can be made to any time length, although blank commercially available cassettes are standardised at 30 minutes, 60 minutes, 90 minutes, etc.

Over the last few years, the quality of portable audio cassette recording equipment has improved enormously. In the past, poor microphone quality and inability to manipulate the signal being recorded meant that it was unlikely to provide a master which would be suitable for reproduction. Using the better quality new generation of this equipment makes audio-recording more accessible to the educational provider without a large budget, but creating an instant master in this way brings its own restrictions, editing the result can be very difficult, and there is less freedom to manipulate the contents to optimise the educational value.

Computers

There is not space here to cover fully the physical characteristics of computers, and the subject needs to be broken down into the origination of the materials (data capture) and the ways in which computers can be used by the student. And any description of computer and video based systems as a series of discrete entities is somewhat artificial since converging technologies have brought the technical possibility of digitising almost anything that moves! Hardware and software choices both for origination and dissemination are constrained more by resource implications than by available technology.

Computer based learning (CBL) can be produced using a standard PC-based set-up consisting of disk drive, CPU, and screen together with commercially available authoring software. Some authoring systems demand very little from the author in terms of computing knowledge beyond basic keyboard skills, but authoring software which can be used to produce stimulating learning by using all available facilities may demand more technical expertise. There are also dedicated integrated hardware and software authoring/delivery systems available.

Sophistication of authoring software is constrained by the capabilities of the hardware, but provides a framework for the originator to present the subject material using predetermined routes and branches which provide opportunities for the learner to interact with the material. A 'lesson' can thus be originated and stored on disk, reproduced and distributed to the students or learning centre. It might also be made available through a networked system, or by modem link to a mainframe computer from remote terminals. Again, the 'product quality' of materials will be constrained by the capabilities of the computers being used by both author and user, but this can reach a very high quality of integrated text and graphics, and can incorporate external material which has been digitised by scanning techniques and inserted wholesale into the learning materials. If printer facilities are available to the learner, the material can also be output to provide hard copy.

Video

Despite a multiplicity of end-uses, originating a video involves a camera, microphone, a recorder/player, videotape and preferably a monitor of some kind. The process involves capturing signals from camera and microphone on magnetic tape, via a VCR (Video Camera Recorder) which can also be used to display and replay the recording through a monitor (screen). The magnetic tape can then be edited by playing the signal back and re-recording selected sequences onto a second tape to provide a master. The image can be manipulated by feeding the signal through a vision-mixer to create special effects and text can be computer-generated and fed through the mixer to be added as captions to the image stored on the master. Reproduction involves high-speed dubbing or digitising technology. Unfortunately, this is where simplicity ends! In addition to international variation and incompatibilities of each of the physical components involved, different professional and domestic systems exist in Britain (eg Betamax, VHS, U-Matic) which may affect the suitability of the video for reproduction purposes although it may be adequate for domestic use.

The cost of video programmes is a product of the level of sophistication of the programme, or 'value added' in terms of the number of people required to plan, produce and record the material, and the specialised techniques and time required to edit it. Traditionally, linear video and broadcast television is very demanding in terms of these 'production values' and hence is very expensive to produce.

Interactive video

Interactive video (IV) systems involve the use of both computer and video to deliver the material and may be tape or disc based. The computer and video player communicate via a 'black-box' and output to the same screen. Viewed either as an enhancement for computer based learning or as an enhancement of video based learning, interactive video is essentially a harnessing of the two technologies, using the computer both to drive the video sequences and to provide the CBL sequences. Interactivity is provided by the learners using a keyboard, keypad, or a touch sensitive monitor screen to move to another sequence or to respond to a stimulus. Some IV systems also provide the means of recording such learning responses.

Tape-based systems use a video tape which has a pre-recorded series of electronic pulses at one-second intervals which provides the specific points of reference to be utilised by the computer to automatically locate any position on the tape. The video sequences are then dubbed onto a different channel. CBL techniques can then be used to create the learning session. IV authoring software exists for this purpose which allows the author to specify whether the sequence originates from the video tape or from the computer (eg CAVIS, FELIX, MENTOR). Tape-based IV tends to be somewhat unwieldy, simply because of the time taken by the video player to locate the correct frame to start a sequence, which can take several seconds if the learning sequence involves complex branches or loops. While freeze-frame and slow motion playback are possible, they are somewhat unsatisfactory.

Many of the physical deficiencies of tape-based IV are overcome by interactive videodisc technology - at a cost. An optical disk substitutes for tape in providing images from a laser-read disk. Learning sequences are first recorded on film or broadcast quality videotape, and are then transferred to a master videodisc usiɳg a laser-based photochemical process which makes an exact copy of the original images and sounds.

Telecommunication

Broadly speaking, telecommunications encompasses any electronic data communications using broadcast, cable or satellite. The last decade has seen a number of educational initiatives utilising such communications, such as teletext (eg ORACLE, CEEFAX), viewdata (PRESTEL, OPTEL), and remote conferencing (CYCLOPS).

In the preparation of teletext material, computer hardware and software are used to create 'pages' of information, some of these pages being reserved for indexing purposes to allow the user to find the required information quickly. These pages are coded and then transmitted in a continuous cyclical stream of four per second, the maximum recommended pages being 100 to prevent lengthy time delays for the user when jumping to different sections of information. Many modern television sets are equipped to receive, decode and display CEEFAX information, accessed through a remote keypad. Apart from allowing the user to select appropriate information and hold a page on screen for as long as desired, it is possible for the transmitted signal stored on disk or magnetic tape for subsequent local generation of hard copy; however, this is still a very passive and one-way form of communication. Originating and amending CEEFAX material is not costly, but broadcasting demands a dedicated frequency, and users need at least an appropriate television receiver and preferably a modified microcomputer.

Given the physical limitations of teletext and its restricted educational potential, it is not surprising that educators prefer to concentrate on developments in the field of viewdata technology, such as PRESTEL.
Like CBL and teletext, material is developed using computer hardware and authoring software, but the data is accessed via the public telephone network and a decoder modem rather than broadcast as a coded signal. Data can be screened passively on a television receiver like teletext, or can be linked a computer. In the latter case, because communication is essentially computer-to-computer, more selectivity and potential interactivity is inherently available but there are a number of additional advantages, not least of which is the possibility of accessing large encyclopaedic databases. Viewdata can be used to provide a public information network like PRESTEL, a national or

local subscriber network of specialised information, such as share dealings, or in-house facilities for message distribution or information. Data can also be retrieved and stored on a local terminal, so viewdata can also be used to transmit computer programmes or provide local hard copy. Micronet 800, for instance, provides a telesoft service available by subscription via a viewdata network. The public telephone network can be used to route subscribers to their own viewdata system (via gateways) and so offer the educational user an attractive means of communicating and disseminating information very quickly. As well as transmitting 'pages' of text and graphics, viewdata technology has the capacity to transmit moving images, this use being known as videotext. Videotext can allow gateway users access to a range of facilities through the public network, including interactive video and CBL material. If used for courseware, origination costs for viewdata need not be any more expensive than CBL, but it is arguable whether a viewdata system has any advantages over a dedicated CBL system using a mainframe computer with remote terminals running on a time-share basis, especially given the subscriber hardware costs and operating expenses incurred with viewdata.

The public telephone network can also be utilised for teleconferencing, although it is also possible to install a private network. Teleconferencing can be used for multi-way communication of anything which can be converted to an electronic signal and conveyed down a telephone line in real time. A teleconferencing session is booked for a pre-arranged time slot and involves a conference bridge being provided as a dial in operator linked service, for dedicated telephone handset or a loudspeaking telephone at a study centre which allows all users simultaneous access to communicate with each other.

Generally speaking, telecommunication technology is not readily accessible to small educational providers unless they can piggy-back onto existing networks or can form consortia with other providers. The initial investment of time and money is one negative factor, the other being the continuing organisational and operational demands once the system is in operation.

Media in action

The contribution of media to any particular course will depend on a number of factors such as the course objectives, structures, students, etc. However, each medium has particular intrinsic properties which make it most suitable for creating particular learning opportunities.

Using audio-tape

Audio-tape is a highly convenient and relatively inexpensive medium which is particularly useful for providing individualised instruction. It can use many of the 'dramatic' motivational techniques of TV, but it is more accessible for learners. Bates (1982) concludes that the greatest media development achievement of the Open University has been the development of the audio-cassette. As with print, audio-cassettes offer the learner individual control and flexibility of use; however, unlike print, audio-tape can convey stress and inflexion and thereby the enthusiasm and interest of the speaker. It can be used for the presentation of music, dialects and social interactions, and this latter facility may become increasingly useful for the exploration of communication in nursing.

A graphic illustration of the impact of audio-tape is provided in an account in Stainton Rogers (1987) of using a recording made by a woman caring for her elderly mother. One student, a head of an old people's home, was profoundly affected by hearing the tape and subsequently changed the policy in the home to involve carers much more in the care of relatives. The student's explanation makes the point:

> To make the change, I had to know how it felt to be a daughter, I had to see the behaviour in terms of what it felt like to be her. It was hearing a real person, all the emotion in her voice, hearing her crying and describing breaking point. It was that which convinced me.
>
> Stainton Rogers 1987

Because it can convey intimacy, Ryan (1987) suggests that audio-cassettes can be useful in supporting the learner as well as carrying the 'taught' component of a course. A teacher can easily record a 'chat' about, for example, difficult aspects of the course or problems with an assignment, which can readily be reproduced and sent to a group of learners.

TV/video

Bates (1987) considers that television has two main strengths in promoting learning. First, it can show material not otherwise available; it might be inaccessible because of geographical distance or because the students would not be allowed access or because it does not exist in the real world. Details of physiology, for example, can be shown either by giving a 'microscope view' or by the use of animation and graphics. Social situations which are unfamiliar to students, such as mourning rituals, can be shown. Second, it can relate theory to practice by giving concrete examples of abstract principles.

However, there is also a very basic level of using video within education: TVI (Tutored-Video Instruction). This can be used as a means of providing learners with lecture type material simply by recording subject specialists using blackboard-and-chalk presentations and delivering the lesson with camera and recorder as their audience. Presentations can be made more attractive to the viewer by editing the material to include other information or graphics.

All linear programmes, however, do involve a passive learning situation; they do not allow for interaction between medium and learner, although the learner may, of course be given a task to complete either while viewing or immediately afterwards in order to focus attention on key elements. As with any medium learners need to be helped to utilise its full potential, and the danger is that 'because television is such a familiar medium, it tends to be taken for granted that students will know how to learn from it. This is not the case' (Bates 1987). Students need help, which can be built into the programme and provided as support to turn the experience from a passive one to an active one.

Computer Based Learning

Computer based learning (CBL) is an umbrella term which includes any way of using computers in education and training (Laurillard 1987). Other terms are computer assisted learning (CAL) which refers mainly to educational programmes run on computers, and computer based training (CBT) which is a term mainly used in industry and can include training for word-processing and other computer skills which, almost by definition, would require a computer base. CBL can provide a high degree of interaction between student and system, guiding the learner through relevant materials at her own pace. Indeed, the student is forced by the medium to interact with the equipment. Text and graphics can be easily combined, and sophisticated equipment allows for the inclusion of animated graphics, photographic stills and moving images. The capacity of CBL to deliver simulation allows the student to develop solutions and strategies without the cost and danger of acquiring these in real life. A by-product is obviously the development of the cognitive skills required simply to operate the equipment!

The disadvantages of CBL are that it can restrict the range and richness of learning experiences because, while it is self-pacing and provides a variety of routes through the learning, those routes are pre-defined and highly structured and thus are unlikely to be suitable for affective learning. Many educational programmes mimic the page-turning characteristics of text-based learning and Laurillard (1987) suggests that a useful question to ask is: 'Couldn't you do the same thing more efficiently with a text (video/workbook, etc.)?

However, another use for computers in open learning is to provide an encyclopaedic knowledge database which can be interrogated in a number of ways ('knowledge-based' or 'expert-systems'). As these are generally (but not necessarily) unsuitable for traditional computer learning programmes, they are more commonly used as part of more complex courseware such as video-tex or video-disk based courseware. Such courseware is very demanding in terms of developmental costs and effort. CBL is itself very expensive to develop; one hears of ratios of development time to course duration of between 100-150:1.

Computer mediated communication

Using a computer to communicate can take various forms, such as electronic mail or computer conferencing, and is potentially important as a remedy for the problem of the slow speed of communication within a distance teaching system using post. While the telephone is as quicker, or quicker if the callers are accessible, it does not usually supply a written record as a computer will. The idea of electronic mail was investigated in the mid-1980s by a number of Open Tech projects, including the Distance Learning Centre, which did not proceed with it because so few nurses would have access to a personal computer. However, more recent work within the Dutch Open University (van Meurs and Bohuijs 1989) indicates that it reduces flexibility of place in studying and adds a dimension of technical difficulty:

> The implementation of a comprehensive system was certainly a technical achievement, but the vulnerability of the various components was evident, and no educational advantages of a tele-education approach over a standard distance-education course could be detected.
>
> van Meurs and Bouhuijs 1989

Interactive video

Interactive video is a technology still in its infancy and the production remains costly. The promise of real interactivity is high as so many alternative routes through the material can be made available at speed, and there is potential for learning decision making skills. However, because of the cost and the inaccessibility to the learner it would be indicated only for specific and complex learning needs (Bates 1987).

Media selection

Bates (1982) suggests a five point guideline for choosing media:

- accessibility - is it available in students' homes
- convenience - can the student use the medium
- academic control - can the teacher design the material herself
- 'human' touch - can the learner relate to the teacher via the medium
- availability - what is available now.

However, there are also a number of practical considerations that need to be borne in mind; trade-offs are complex and can sometimes be unique to a particular organisation. The three major considerations are educational, financial and political.

Financial considerations may themselves be complex. Take labour costs, for example, which constitute a major cost element in the development of open learning materials. These are a critical cost factor if full-time expertise needs to be bought in from outside the organisation, but may reduce significantly if existing staff are seconded to a project for fixed time periods. Similarly, a medium which in the short term may involve relatively large origination costs may be less costly to reproduce or to update than other media (eg CBT v print). This economic information involves at least the following:

- the capital costs of establishing delivery systems
- the capital costs of any materials development systems required
- the recurrent costs of operating these systems (salaries, overheads, etc.)
- which of the above costs will be fixed and which will be variable
- cost-benefit information (eg potential savings in other areas)
- economic operating criteria, such as 'Will this system be subsidised or self financing?'

In addition to this 'hard' financial information, cost-effectiveness information is required, which must be closely related to the providers goals. Thus the choice between one medium and another must also address the goals; one such might be to extend learning opportunities to new students, another might be to contribute towards the quality of the learning experience, or to overcome teacher shortages in specialised areas, and so on.

Until relatively recently, educational economics and organisation tolerated classroom based learning, with relatively short course development saving time at the cost of duplication of effort (ie a number of different teachers involved in the same course at different geographical locations). A shift towards open learning brings a need almost to reverse the traditional approach towards the development and organisation of education. There is a need both to understand educational requirements well in advance and to concentrate the resources for ensuring the educational options for meeting those requirements and for implementing the choices made as a result. This implies a requirement for specialist centres for the staff and technical resources involved in the planning, provision and delivery of educational and training materials for nursing.

Media decisions are also dictated by potential student populations. Those media which are expensive to produce may still compare favourably with other educational methods in terms of cost-per-student where you have a large student population.

The exploitation of media in nurse education

In nursing education the exploitation of media within open learning has only just begun and therefore there are few precedents to guide choices. However, the Open University has successfully mixed video, audio-cassette and print in P553 *A Systematic Approach to Nursing Care* (Open University 1984) and, although in general it has been a successful package involving both group and individual work, it could be said that the print based material has stood the test of time rather better than the video. Neither of the two Open Tech projects (Distance Learning Centre and Continuing Nurse Education) had a budget for making videos, but the Distance Learning Centre (DLC) has incorporated audio-cassettes into some of their learning materials. Some of the audiotapes made for the Diploma in Nursing course were made cheaply and simply using widely available cassette tape recorders to interview various people on their opinions about nursing. While the sound quality is not good, these tapes do carry an immediate impact and offer an addition learning dimension to the student on what is a long, and doubtless inevitably wearisome, three year journey.

However, the inclusion of audio-tapes in the independent learning packs of the Managing Care series illustrates the small but significant problem of storing such materials. If the packs are sold directly to a learner then storage is unlikely to be a problem, and at the other end of the spectrum a properly equipped resource centre is unlikely to experience difficulties. Ordinary libraries, however, can find it difficult to store 'packs' of material in spaces designed for books and difficult to monitor 'wear and tear' on non-print components, and at least one library has abandoned the use of all but the print components of the pack.

Perhaps the most important initiative in nurse education which explored complex media was the Nightingale School Computer Assisted Learning Project. This project aimed to explore the use of Computer Assisted Learning (CAL) as a teaching and learning resource for the promotion of nursing competencies. The project, which produced and evaluated a CAL package for learning IV drug administration, produced two major conclusions. First, that CAL as an educational methodology was acceptable within nursing and was in practice highly motivating for the students. Second, that successful integration of CAL in nurse education depends on a high level of quality of product and a high level of competence amongst the teachers (Norman *et al* 1988). These conclusions could, of course, be applied to any medium and any area of open learning, but are perhaps particularly welcome within CAL where enthusiasm for the medium sometimes gets in the way of careful evaluation of its results. The conclusions of the project are in part being followed up by the ENB CAL project which aims to help teachers acquire skills in educational information technology (ENB 1987).

Exciting though the possibilities of new technology are in education, the comments of the RCN on the ENB CAL programme add an air of realism:

> Within the framework, the inclusion of the research component is essential in order to monitor and evaluate the consequences of this new technology to what must be regarded as quite a traditional learning setting.
> ...Quite clearly, the training programme required to bring existing nurse teachers to the state of being computer 'literate' will be a major undertaking, particularly in the light of the shortage of them and the pressures of work to which they are subjected.
>
> RCN 1987

Within nursing the impact of the new educational technologies will relate to at least three factors. First, the type and quality of production, second, the teacher's skills in supporting the learners using the technology and third, the utility of each of the technologies to the goals of nurse education. Enthusiasts for one or other of the technologies are not always best placed to think through the complex trade-offs of costs and benefits essential before major investments are made. Enthusiasts are often keen on the production side rather than the support of the learner and an important message coming from many of the proponents of new technology (*see*, for example, Bates 1987 and Laurillard 1987) is that production needs a very large central investment. The challenge at the local level may be to define educational goals in such a way that producers can meet the criteria laid down.

References

Bates A 1982 Trends in the use of audio-visual media. In Daniel J et al *Learning at a Distance.* ICCE Edmonton

Bates A W 1987 Learning from television. In Thorpe M and Grugeon D (eds.) *Open Learning for Adults.* Longman

Duchastel P C 1988 Designing intelligent learning environments. In Mathias H, Rushby N, Budgett R (eds) Aspects of Educational Technology No21 *Designing New Systems and Technologies For Learning.* Kogan Page

ENB 1987 *CAL Project Report.* English National Board

Keegan D 1986 *The Foundations of Distance Education.* Croom Helm

Knowles M 1984 *The Adult Learner: a Neglected Species.* Gulf Publishing Co.

Laurillard D 1987 Introducing computer-based learning. In Thorpe M and Grugeon D (eds) *Open Learning For Adults.* Longman

Norman S E, Chapman E J, Hinton T 1988 The Nightingale School Computer Assisted Learning Projects. University of Surrey

Open University 1984 *A Systematic Approach to Nursing Care.* The Open University Press

Ryan S 1987 Using audio-tape to support the learner. In Thorpe M and Grugeon D (eds.) *Open Learning for Adults.* Longman

RCN 1987 Comments on: *A Framework for the development of CAL for Nurses Midwives and Health Visitors* (Draft ENB Oct 1986). Royal College of Nursing

Stainton Rogers W 1987 Adapting materials for alternative use. In Thorpe M and Grugeon D (eds.) *Open Learning for Adults.* Longman

van Meurs C E J and Bouhuijs P A J 1989 Tele-education: an experiment on home computing at the Dutch Open University *Open Learning* 4 1 pp33-6

Part 3:
The ecstasy of delivery

9 Delivering open learning: an overview

Kate Robinson

The existence of open learning materials alone does not constitute an open learning system. At the very least, potential learners have to be informed about the existence of the materials and the administrative arrangements for acquiring them. However, there is potentially much more than this to an open learning delivery system. Ideally the system delivers not just a piece of hardware – a text, videotape or whatever – but an educational experience. This experience may vary from a full-time degree course to the study of a short package of learning materials, and the support provided in each case may be radically different. Subsequent chapters will look at some particular examples of support systems, but there are some general principles and problems which can be examined here.

What, then, is meant by *delivery*? An overall definition might be that it is the system which enables the learner to use the learning materials in an efficient and effective way. The support system is not something that is tacked onto the the interaction between the learner and the learning material. It does not 'make up for' the deficiencies of the materials, and neither does it 'do the things materials cannot do'; it enhances the whole learning experience of the individual. Support is usually delivered by a human agency but in some cases it is technology based, as in computer feedback on assignments, for example, or computer tutorials (Open University 1988). However, it is the human element which is usually paramount and the following discussion will look at possible roles and necessary skills, and the sort of structures within which teachers and others can interact with the learner.

Roles

The use of a learning package means that one part of the teaching role has been 'locked away' and does not need to be serviced. In general the learning materials will deal with the subject area or specific competencies rather than general counselling, guidance and study skills. This is not an absolute distinction and materials can also offer guidance on study skills and related life-skills, but in general the role assigned to the 'human' part of the system is related to the individualised counselling and helping which is often known by the umbrella term of *guidance*. Within the Open Tech context *guidance* was defined (Bailey 1987b) as:

- *informing* – the learner of everything she needs to know at a suitable time and in a suitable form;
- *advising* – the learner on appropriate ways forward based on the teacher's greater experience and knowledge;
- *counselling* – the learner in a non-directive way to help her explore her own potential and make appropriate choices;
- *coaching* – the learner by providing learning situations which will enhance her progress;
- *assessment* – of the learner in all her capacities and sharing that information with her;
- *advocacy* – on behalf of the learner in order to remove obstacles to learning.

These activities are required by individual learners at different stages in their learning 'career', and within open learning there is perhaps more emphasis on the idea of helping the learner through the whole process of learning, beginning with pre-entry, continuing through enrolment and the study of the course and finishing with the exit process.

Combining the idea of a learner career with a set of necessary guidance skills produces a matrix of activities such as is presented in Figure 9.1 (Bailey 1987a). The matrix also includes two important sets of activities beyond guidance and within evaluation - feedback and assessment.

This matrix defines what can be offered to the learner, not what she may necessarily need, or want, to accept. There is some discussion about whether support should be offered proactively or reactively. Rumble (1989) contrasts the policy of the Open University, which considers that support needs to be proactive to prevent failure and promote success, with the policy of the West German Fern Universität which sees proactive intervention as an erosion of learner independence and an invasion of privacy.

The activities described above can, and perhaps should, be split between a number of people, working in a number of roles, which may have different titles in different institutions.

	Informing	Advising	Counselling	Coaching	Advocacy	Feedback to systems	Assessment
PRE ENTRY	– range of options – finance – OL scheme details – company intentions	– levels of difficulty – need for preparation – pros and cons of OL – job prospects	– reviewing needs – awareness raising – appraising current work role – coping with blocks	– decision making	– employer contacts OL scheme for employee – guidance helper contacts scheme for client – scheme contacts LEA on fees	– by OL scheme to companies on training needs – to funding agencies on grants	– formal aptitude tests – self-diagnosis of capabilities
ENROLMENT	– specific details on packages, practicals, tutorials, methods of payment	– study skills – order of modules	– choosing a programme – understanding OL – boosting confidence	– learning management skills	– scheme approaches employer about time off, fees, support – helpers contact careers service etc. on job prospects	– to validating bodies on credit exemptions	– informal (vocational) assessment
ON LEARNING	– use of libraries – update of modules available – whereabouts of other learners	– where to study – who can help	– using assessment constructively – learning styles – coping with blocks	– running self-help groups – planning time – using telephone support – handling self-assessment questions	– referral to counsellor or guidance specialist – liaison with employer/trainer	– from employer on work performance – to MSC on gaps in provision – to colleges/employers on OL	– range of assessment from: tutor, trainer, peer, self
EXIT	– new range of learning options – data on jobs	– where to get specialist help next	– appraisal of current position – exploration of new needs	– writing up reports – applying learning to workplace practice – self-preservation	– referral for further training – liaison with Jobcentre or careers service	– to/from guidance agencies on OL as a form of training – to employers' bodies	– reprofiling – final assessment

Figure 9.1 Matrix of activities

Tutor
A tutor will have expertise in the specialist subject area and in promoting and assessing the knowledge and skills involved in the course. She will be familiar with the ideas, concepts and language of the course and with where they are likely to cause difficulty. She will also have generic skills such as giving advice, running groups, etc.

Counsellor
Unlike the tutor, the counsellor need not have subject expertise. She will, however, understand the learning process and be skilled at promoting learning at individual and group levels. She may also be able to negotiate within the relevant organisations on behalf of the learner - or at least give appropriate advice. For reasons which will be discussed below, the two roles of tutor and counsellor are sometimes put together.

Mentor
An additional common role in vocational education is that of the mentor, who is typically employed in the same organisation as the learner, although often in a capacity with more access to resources than the learner. She guides the learner in applying the new knowledge in a practical fashion within the workplace. She will help the learner as an individual learn from practise and place that learning in a framework which will link it to other aspects of the learner's work. She may have more specialised or up-to-date practical knowledge than the tutor, and she may also be able to help within negotiating with the organisation for access or resources necessary to the learner.

However, there is another part of the mentor role which is not vocationally based and which is concerned with encouraging and motivating the student, and this can be performed by almost anyone. In establishing a support network for open learners we probably underestimate the help that is given to them by friends and family – a consequence of seeing learners in classroom situations rather than in their home environment. This help could be channelled constructively if it was acknowledged and discussed more openly, and learners could be helped to choose and use such mentors. Similarly, other learners provide encouragement and reassurance and, within a vocational programme, a wealth of experience to draw on.

Skills

Supporting open learners requires particular skills, but the precise nature of them depends on whether the support is organised on an individual or a group basis and whether there is any face-to-face contact. However, despite the differences the idea of 'learner-centredness' provides a consistent theme; the focus of the support is the learner and not the subject. Obviously this concept is not unique to open learning, but it does assume a new prominence because the learning materials will have taken over much of the traditional teaching role.

Teaching at a distance

Teaching at a distance usually involves a one-to-one relationship between teacher and learner, which, because of the distance factor, will be unusual. First, it is not mediated through a group, and second, it may have to be sustained in a relationship in which teacher and learner never meet. The context of the learner is more obviously family or work relationships rather then a group of learners isolated from their 'normal' context. This allows a close relationship, provided the teacher focuses on the learner and not the materials. The temptation is to see the role as facilitating the author of the materials to get the message across by, for example, explaining difficult passages or adding new material, rather than facilitating the learner to get the most out of the material. Obviously there may be times when there is an error or omission in the materials which deserves attention but, in general, work should be dictated by the individual learner's problems with their learning.

There are a number of specific skills which will help a learner get the most out of their experience and avoid compromising the control of the learner over the time, pace and place of their learning. For example, teaching by post and telephone allows issues to be dealt with according to the learner's timetable. However, teaching on the telephone is not an easy skill. Learners will often present their problems either in terms of the text -'I can't understand page 46' - or in terms of their own inadequacies – 'I can't cope with this course, at all.' The teacher needs the skill to focus on the particular learning process in which the individual has got 'stuck' and to negotiate a way out which the learner can manage. If control is to remain with the learner then they must be helped to diagnose their own problems rather than become dependent on support from the teacher. As Northedge (1987) summarises the process:

> Very little advice on specific practices suits everyone and all circumstances. In the end individual students have to be able to guide themselves by trial and error and reflection and experience... advice should press in the direction of *exploration* and *self-reflection...*

In some systems teachers use teleconferencing facilities to conduct group work at a distance and there are particular skills attached to this which need to be acquired by both teacher and learners. Computers also enable tutors to communicate with a group.

Marking assignments
The technique of marking assignments at a distance from the learner also requires particular expertise to ward off the dangers of ambiguity and de-motivation. The Open University has done a great deal of research in this area and monitors the marking of its tutors to ensure that they offer constructive and detailed feedback to the students. However, the important principle is to remember that one of the functions of the assessment process is to form a relationship with the learner rather than with the written assignment. Comments should relate to the learner and should reflect the status of the written answers as part of the learning process of an individual in particular circumstances rather than as an acontextual product to be judged (Miers 1987; Sewart 1987). The judging process may be necessary within the context of a formally assessed course, but it is not the central concern of the teacher in the process.

Mediating
Within the Open University the role of the tutor-counsellor as intermediary between the student and the institution has been discussed (Miers 1987) but in vocational education there is another mediating role – that of intermediary between learner and employer. The teacher needs to ensure that the learner is in the best possible position to gain from their learning experience in terms of, for example, putting new ideas into practice, participating in new ways of organising work and exploring new techniques. Such experiences may be inhibited by the constraints of operating the service and the intermediary has to explore the middle ground between the needs of the learners and of the service. This kind of activity is often best performed by a workplace mentor rather than a tutor or counsellor from outside the organisation.

Group work

Although open learning should focus on the individual, the reality is that in some systems many teachers only meet their learners within the context of a group. P553 *A Systematic Approach to Nursing Care* (Open University 1984), for example, is usually studied within the framework of eight group sessions which are facilitated by a teacher or manager. These sessions help the learners consolidate their learning and provide a forum in which they can discuss what change is possible in their work environment. Such groups are difficult to facilitate, not least because the constraints of work and staggered holiday times may prevent a consistent group being maintained across a lengthy series of sessions. The groups are also often very mixed in ability, both academic and clinical, and in clinical background, so forging common links yet maintaining the importance of each individual's learning is a challenge.

Evidence from the Open University system where the role of group tutorials has been closely studied (and hotly debated) shows that learners bring a wide range of expectations and needs to the tutorial (Kelly 1987). Often the learner's expectations of such a group reflect their experience of conventional teaching rather than open learning and the teacher may have to work hard to wean them from such dependence. There is a danger of the learner getting 'mixed messages' if the group sessions within an open learning system are teacher centred rather than learner centred.

Structures

Constructing a support system within an existing institution is complex and difficult. The Open University had the great advantage of building in a 'green field' environment, but setting up an open learning support system within an existing institution means fitting into existing methods of working, staff roles and union agreements. To do this successfully may require that a senior member of staff is responsible to give advice and guide the innovation (Dixon 1987).

The structures which are established should reflect the roles which need to be filled and the skills available. For example, it is important to consider whether the support structure should be linked to:

- a particular course or study programme
- an individual learner
- a workplace environment.

If the focus is on the learner's individual difficulties then it follows that the support structure should aim to form lasting pairings between learner and teacher. However, there are logistical and academic reasons why this might not be possible. For example, if the teacher and learner are sister and staff nurse working together on a ward, should or could this pairing continue if either changes jobs? Similarly, some courses, such as assertive skills, may present the learner with particular difficulties which some teachers are better at resolving than others. The inevitable tensions between the different requirements need to be worked out in particular contexts, and a number of models are working successfully in assessed open learning schemes although we know less about the support of unassessed local schemes. The Open University, for example, has a system of tutor-counsellors who provide all the necessary support to their students in their foundation studies, but in subsequent years the role is split and a subject specialist takes on the tutoring aspects while the tutor-counsellor retains the counselling function. This allows for both continuity within the system – a student would usually have the same tutor-counsellor throughout their degree programme – but also provides, via the specialist tutor, the students with the expertise needed for each individual course. Within the Open University system this is particularly important as tutors also mark assignments, but the formal assessment function can be separated out and given to an assessor, as it is in the DLC Diploma in Nursing system (these systems are explored further in Chapter 11).

Once decisions have been taken about who will fill the various roles described above, it is important to decide what training they require and how their existing job descriptions may need to be changed. An important issue is determining the workload of the support staff. Forward planning of classroom teaching is relatively simple in as much as you can predict the length of time devoted to teaching, you can guess at the amount of preparation time (the accepted ratio is about 1:1) and you know that individual queries arising from the groupwork will be automatically constrained by the amount of time you are not available because you are teaching elsewhere. However, teaching a group of open learning students requires predictions about what work this caseload will generate, both in terms of offering open workshops, that is, times when the learners may study on the premises and use the resources, including a teacher, and individual telephone, post and face to face tuition.

Management and administrative support

Conventional teaching has traditionally received very little administrative support, but it is a vital element in open learning. The existence of constraints means that people's activities are generally predictable; the removal of those constraints in an open learning system means that activities are unpredictable and need to be monitored much more closely. For example, for learning materials to be available to learners when they need them either large stocks must be held, which is prohibitively expensive, or the movement of stocks must be closely monitored and use negotiated with individual learners. Similarly, if assessment is not at fixed times then the administrative burden of keeping assignments secure and keeping records of the learner's progress increases dramatically. So much so that, although the existence of learning materials makes an individual roll-on, roll-off system within a formal, assessed course possible, the accompanying administrative problems make them very rare. For an open learning system of any complexity a computer record facility is essential.

Physical resources

Although open learning does not in general take place in classrooms it does not follow that learners do not need physical resources. These include quiet rooms for study, rooms for support group or tutorial meetings and access to suitable equipment. Within the Open University system the local study centres (established throughout the country in local colleges) were intended to provide space for individual and group study as well as formal tutorial sessions, but in practice they have rarely been used for this – students preferring to view television programmes at home, and group meetings happening as often as not in the pub. Nevertheless, space should be provided as not all learners have home situations conducive to studying.

Supporting learners in the workplace

The motivation for adults to become involved in open learning varies enormously and many do so for the sheer excitement of learning. However, others take courses because of their working situation - either to improve their qualifications in order to change their work or to improve their competency to do their current job. This latter group forms a large part of continuing education in nursing and therefore of the potential users of open learning. However, they may have particular problems which require particular forms of guidance (Bailey 1988), although the basic aims of guidance are similar to those in other situations:

- to clarify and strengthen the learner's motivation
- to improve the relevance of learning
- to improve the quality of learning

The problems arise in vocational education partly from the interrelationship of organisation and individual goals which may become more problematic as the learning moves away from a simple training model towards empowering the learner not just to dictate her own learning pattern and also to create a dialogue between the concepts learned and her practice situation. If the learner is to achieve real learning, she will have to try the concepts out in the workplace, and thereby challenge the existing practice within the work situation. P553 *A Systematic Approach to Nursing Care* (Open University 1984), for example, talks about partnership with the patient, which requires a new way of approaching and negotiating with each client, not just minor amendments to details of practice routine. The guidance role in this situation must involve mediation between the learner and the organisation as well as individual support to the learner. This may be problematic in a situation in which the person giving guidance is also a member of the organisation and subject to particular constraints of her own.

A workplace network

A network of guidance facilities within a workplace would offer all learners open learning resources when required. Such a network can be of various complexities and demand various resources. Bailey (1988) suggests four dimensions of planning:

- the level and comprehensiveness of the system
- whether it should be proactive or reactive
- the integration with other learning elements
- the range of resources used

But whatever the level of resource devoted to the system it should reflect the characteristics of the workplace situation, for example whether learners are scattered or grouped, whether the learners form a homogeneous or heterogeneous group, etc. And it should receive some degree of management commitment, not least because the line managers may form an important part of the support network and need to have the necessary investment of time recognised. However, two other possible sources of support may be more important than in a general learning situation - first the use of peer groups, and second the creation of resource centres.

Peer groups

Peer groups or action learning circles (Bailey 1988) can be formed as part of the group work arranged around an open learning pack such as P553 *A Systematic Approach to Nursing Care* (Open University 1984). In a survey of the function of group work connected to three different learning packs for health care workers, Grant notes:

> The group environment can be used to advantage to help students to realise the practical possibilities for change in their own professional practice by planning the introduction of changes and developments, discussing these with peers in the group to ascertain their views of feasibility and making a commitment to the implementation of change that is supported by the group.
>
> Grant 1987

Of course, for work such as nursing which essentially involves interaction and negotiation, the experience of the group is itself a useful learning experience.

Resource centres

Within a vocational scheme it is important for resources to be made available at work; that is one way in which the employer can make a positive statement of commitment and encouragement. For nurses it is particularly important because their working environment often precludes taking advantage of resources in the community. A self-help group of learners on night duty, for example, are hardly in a position to go to the pub in their break.

Ideally an open learning centre should be set up incorporating a library of materials and an information service, perhaps using one of the computer databases of learning opportunities such as MARIS-NET. It would offer use of equipment such as tape recorders, video-players, and televisions in a friendly and comfortable environment. Open learning teachers can use such a centre as a base, particularly if it incorporates small rooms for individual counselling and for group work. Evidence from industry (Greenacre 1987; Cox and Hobson 1988) suggests that such centres are well used by the workforce for both vocational *and* general education.

One of the problems of the health service, however, is the dispersal of the workforce, so an outreach capacity is essential. Again an ideal would be an 'open learning bus' supplying a number of small centres around the periphery of a district and also offering facilities to the isolated nurses in health centres and small hospitals.

The nursing context

Despite the well documented evidence of the importance of coherent effective support, there is no evidence from an extensive survey of open learning (Lawrence *et al* 1988) that effective support networks exist within nurse education other than those attached to particular courses such as the Diploma in Nursing by distance learning. Moreover, they found that many teachers who were involved in open learning were concerned about their role:

> Teachers frequently expressed the need for training in the use of distance learning materials and for the development of the facilitator role. There is a sense of anxiety about the loss of control of the learning experience in many of the statements made here by teachers, which may reflect their uncertainty about their own future roles, in particular in participation in distance teaching.
>
> Lawrence *et al* 1988

F

This is in some ways surprising, if only because there seems to be considerable experience of learning through the Open University amongst nurse teachers, and being a learner has been recommended as a way of understanding how to teach within an open learning situation (Miers 1987). Moreover, of the three major difficulties identified (Open Unversity 1988) for teachers in moving from a conventional to an open learning situation

- orienting to education rather than a particular subject
- seeing relationship building as central
- teaching through written comments

at least the first two would seem to also be central to nurse education. Potentially at least, therefore, many of the beliefs and skills appropriate to supporting open learners are already in place in nurse education. The following chapters show how these can be utilised in practical situations.

References

Bailey D 1987a Open learning and guidance, *British Journal of Guidance and Counselling*, 15, 3 pp237-56

Bailey D 1987b *Open Learning and Guidance: a Manual of Practice.* National Institute for Careers Education and Counselling/Manpower Services Commission

Bailey D 1988 Guidance and Counselling in Work-based Open Learning. In Paine N (ed) *Open Learning in Transition.* National Extension College

Cox S and Hobson H 1988 User appreciation of open learning at Jaguar Cars Ltd. *Open Learning*, 3, 1 pp50-52

Dixon K 1987 *Implementing Open Learning in Local Authority Institutions.* Further Education Unit/Open Learning Branch Manpower Services Commission, 2nd edition

Ellington S 1987 The role of the facilitator to an open learning package. Unpublished MA dissertation, Institute of Education, University of London

Grant J 1987 Designing group work for professional updating. In Thorpe M and Grugeon D (eds) *Open Learning for Adults.* Longman

Greenacre L 1987 What is wrong with open learning? *Open Learning*, 2, 3 p41

Kelly P 1987 Tutorial Groups in Open Learning. In Thorpe M and Grugeon D (eds) *Open Learning for Adults.* Longman

Lawrence J, Maggs C, Rogers J 1988 *Interim report on an Evaluation of the Use of Distance Learning Materials for Continuing Professional Education for Qualified Nurses, Midwives and Health Visitors.* Institute of Education, University of London

Miers M 1987 Reflections on the role of correspondence teaching. In Thorpe M and Grugeon D (eds) 1987 *Open Learning for Adults.* Longman

Northedge A 1987 Returning to study. In Thorpe M and Grugeon D (eds) 1987 *Open Learning for Adults.* Longman

Open University 1984 P553 *A Systematic Approach to Nursing Care: an Introduction.* The Open University Press

OU 1988 Open Learning *(D05 Part B/E86 - Module 2, Professional Studies in Post-compulsory Education).* The Open University Press

Rumble G 1989 'Open learning', 'distance learning', and the misuse of language, *Open Learning* 4, 2 pp28-36

Sewart D 1987 Limitations of the learning package. In Thorpe M and Grugeon D (eds) *Open Learning for Adults.* Longman

Thorpe M and Grugeon D (eds) 1987 *Open Learning for Adults* Longman.

10 Supporting learners in the workplace

Steve Wright

> Well, perhaps nobody wanted to come – perhaps they'd all like
> to go – but they're not going... Because they're going to behave
> – and that's what we all have to learn in life – we have to learn
> to behave!
> Ruth Draper *The Children's Party*

Like the exasperated parent in Ruth Draper's story, learning can
produce many dilemmas for both teacher and student. Efforts at open
and distance learning can throw these issues in to sharp focus, for the
requirement of such learning methods puts an emphasis on the learner
determining the process of learning rather than the 'traditional' model
of the teacher led, 'top-down' approach (Hurst 1985).

Current trends in nursing education are placing great emphasis on the
production of the creative, problem-solving practitioner, able to act and
think independently and to employ skills imaginatively (United
Kingdom Central Council 1986). Thus many have argued that a nurse
of this calibre requires lifelong and vigorous educational support of a
type that fosters such creative thinking, for 'creative, problem-solving
nurses' will not be produced *en masse* unless they also have 'creative
nurse teachers and managers' (Wright 1986).

Developing what Dickoff and James (1985) have called the 'thinking-
doer' or what Pearson and Vaughan (1986) have called
'knowledgeable-doers' requires the teachers of nursing not only to be
experts themselves, but also to be the kind of person who can help
learners to help themselves. An educational style of this nature has
become a dominant theme not only in nursing (ENB 1987) but in the
wider field of adult education (Freire 1973; Rogers 1983; Knowles
1984). The implication for such a shift in education patterns should
not be underestimated. Espousing a student-centred philosophy
requires that 'belief in the autonomy of the learner is central, as is the
notion of the teacher as a facilitator of learning rather than an

instructor. These beliefs have a profound effect on the way in which the teacher perceives his or her own role and the way in which the learners perceive the teacher and themselves. Such beliefs also affect notions about the way in which learning should be assessed, and by whom, (ENB 1987).

The challenge for teachers and learners

To support open learning, the first task must therefore be with the teacher, and for some this may require an enormous conceptual leap into a different type of behaviour. For many teachers the adoption of a model of their role as facilitator, resource-person and helper is easy, for others it can be threatening, traumatic or simply unthinkable (Hurst 1985). Thus it is necessary for you, as the teacher, to assess your own approach first and define how you will manage the difficulties and conflicts which may arise. A full debate of this issue is beyond the scope of this text, but many recent writers have produced much useful material for nurse teachers, both on conflict management and self-assessment (Ernst and Goodison 1981; Burns 1983; Burnard 1985; ENB 1987).

If there are difficulties for the teacher in the student-centred approach, then there may be problems for learners. Goodall (1985) notes that students sometimes demand traditional teaching styles, deriving a sense of security from an approach they experienced in school before entering nursing. This, argues Knowles (1984), puts pressure on the teacher to 'tell them what to do'. This is a trap into which both teacher and learner may fall, as they fail to recognise and deal with some of the very real fears that taking charge of your own learning can bring. Knowles goes on to argue that resorting to didactic teaching strategies simply reinforces the learners' dependency and his or her position of inferiority to the teacher. In reality, the students still see themselves as 'adults' having a 'self-concept of being responsible for their own lives', with a 'deep psychological need to be seen by others and treated by others as being capable of self direction. They resent and resist situations in which they feel others are imposing their will on them.' (Knowles 1984).

Rogers (1983) posits that the teacher role is to be 'real, understanding and caring' so that students not only 'learn more of the basics, but exhibit more creativity and problem-solving qualities'. It is indeed, the production of these latter qualities in nursing that is the business of nurse education.

Through open and distance learning, the teacher becomes helper, companion and friend to the learner, encouraging them through a gradual and often difficult process, to take charge of their own lives.

Such 'self-empowerment' (Hopson and Scally 1981) can lead them also to take better control of their own lives. The spinoffs, argue the ENB (1987) are observable:

> Students transfer their learning to other areas of their lives. They become pro-active rather than reactive, anticipating and initiating rather than responding. Teachers who are teaching in this way also become more proactive, more resourceful, more confident, more accepting of themselves and of others, more open to experience and more adaptable when dealing with new situations. They remain learners, understanding that 'the more I know, the more I don't know'. Such wisdom allows honesty in facing limitations, and in looking from the growth point. Such teachers are less judgmental with learners and they find this a liberating experience.
>
> English National Board 1987

There is plenty of evidence to show that what patients want from nurses is creative, effective, caring nursing (Royal Commission 1979; Ombudsman reports 1986/7/8) and that this is what nurses themselves would like to offer (Price Waterhouse 1988; Royal College of Nursing 1986). The challenge of supporting learners in open and distance learning is the challenge of producing excellence in practice.

Some practical measures for helping learners

If we begin with the premise that the first step is for the teacher to critically examine, reappraise and, if necessary, to change their own role in the open learning process, then the next is to identify ways in which the students can be helped to learn for themselves. Adopting self directed learning approaches is not an excuse to abrogate teaching responsibilities and abandon the learners to the knowledge jungle without directions on the means to survive.

In this section, I will draw upon some experiences of myself and my colleagues in supporting students in distance learning as well as examples from relevant literature.

I worked for a long time on a large unit caring for the elderly. It was a big 'workhouse' type setting which had taken on many of the features of what Goffman (1961) would call the 'total institution'. Care had become very ritualised and routinised. Staff were demoralised and disinterested. Resources were poor, the environment depressing. Open learning was to form part of an overall educational strategy to help break the institutional mould. It could be tailor-made to meet certain individual's needs and thus provide one more option, another educational tool. Used with the right staff at the right time, it can help bring challenge and ideas back into nursing.

Resources

A key role for the teacher can be in identifying the resources, facilities and materials the learner may need to pursue their objectives. Having identified these, there may also be a role here for the teacher to actually provide them. The following are some examples:

Access to library/literature facilities
While the students may be aware of some provisions (eg the school of nursing or local libraries) they may need help to gain access to others. The teachers will need to be aware of others (eg university, college or polytechnic libraries), their opening times, the facilities offered and the degree of access available to students who do not belong to these institutions. Some organisations (such as the British Library) organise a postal lending service. Many staff organisations (eg the Royal College of Nursing) provide their members with extensive facilities – including libraries, and help with literature searches. Government departments (eg the Department of Health) and other institutions (eg the Kings Fund Centre) also have considerable literature resources.

Apart from knowing where to direct learners when they come to you for information (incidentally, it is a good idea to keep a catalogue of this for ease of access), it can also be useful to keep a stock of papers, journals and books which you know they will need, especially if you know there may be some difficulty in getting hold of them. Building up your own small scale library for this purpose can be immensely useful. It is also worth considering the special difficulties of night staff – who are likely to have a much more limited opportunity to gain access to the literature. Having the knowledge available 'on site' was, for us, an essential part of our overall strategy to improve care.

> *We set up the nursing library in my office, gradually building up a supply of books that I knew people would ask for. This included taking out regular subscriptions to certain journals. During the day, it's always open. At night, the nursing officer has the key to the office with an understanding that any of the staff can have access to the shelves if needs be. I simply ask the staff to leave me a note of any titles borrowed. It's worked extremely well in practice, and no, we haven't lost a lot of books. Open learning is all about trusting the students after all.*

> Clinical Nurse Specialist

Other learning and project aids
Videos, films, slides and so on, may also form a part of the learner
needs, and the teacher may need to keep a stock of these, or know
where to get them. The clinical specialist mentioned above also kept
video equipment in her office which could be used for a small group of
learners to view particular films. Many learning packages will be
provided with particular videos or other necessary study aids (eg
leaflets, measuring instruments, copies of relevant articles, etc).

From time to time students may have need of typing or photocopying
facilities. Can these be provided with existing resources or can help be
found? The teacher may need to know where such people and
resources are available (and how much they might cost). Learners may
also need access to a telephone to make enquiries, assistance with
postal enquiries or stationery. Another key feature might be the
provision of a quiet room in which to study. I know of one teacher
who made her office available to a student who, because of domestic
circumstances, was having difficulty finding an environment conducive
to study at home. Issues like this in turn lead to the question of funding
(q.v.) to support the learners.

> *Apart from all the lists of libraries and paper that I keep, I
> also have a list of local people with telephone numbers who
> can help with typing and project work, together with how
> much they usually charge.*
>
> Nurse manager

Other individuals and groups
As a teacher, you may be the principal resource person for the learner,
not necessarily giving out all the information yourself, but guiding the
learner as to who and where to go for further information. It is
necessary to identify when other groups (eg research interest groups,
professional organisations, support groups, etc.) are available to help
the learner and where they can be located. Other individuals can also
act as personal tutors offering advice and guidance on a specialised
subject.

> *My studies on cancer nursing led me to seek out several of
> the local specialists in the hospital to pick their brains. My
> tutor helped me out with addresses of specialist hospitals in
> the UK. I wrote to some key people and then was able to
> arrange a visit to one of them.*
>
> Staff Nurse, undertaking research interest course.

Funding
There is great variation in how much learners are supported financially in their studies. Some distance learning material may be quite expensive, and there may be other cost implications (eg pursuing a research study, postage, telephone, typing, travel expenses) involved in some open learning projects. Sometimes these costs can be met from within existing staff training budgets, at other times the learner may be expected to meet all costs themselves. Alternatively, many local and national opportunities exist to seek sponsorship, scholarships and so on which can defer the cost of a course of study. Most settings will seek to supply at least some support to the learners. Purdy and Wright (1986) have identified how they set up a 'nursing bursary' separate from health authority funds to provide additional resources for staff development (eg bulk purchases of distance learning texts), and implemented a variety of measures (eg organising a staff fund raising group, seeking sponsorship, selling expertise outside the health authority) to raise funds to achieve their goals. The use of the bursary in my setting was to be essential in supporting other educational activities; health authorities, after all, having limited funds for this, so the bursary was a useful adjunct – we wished to ensure that no nurse's development was restricted because the money had run out. Having our own bursary separate from health authority funds, gave us far more flexibility to support the staff.

It is useful therefore, for the teacher to be aware of the availability of resources to help learners with their studies, for you will often be the first port of call when help is needed. Sometimes you may be able to provide them yourself (eg help with a few telephone calls, with typing letters or a report) if the scale is within your own resources. Alternatively, you should be able to identify other opportunities. While it could be argued that being prepared to take control of your own learning should also include the learner meeting all the costs themselves, there are many areas where help is essential for those who do not always have such resources. The teacher here can be a vital link in helping to find ways of overcoming inhibitors to learning when these are based solely on grounds of cost.

Tutorials

Both group tutorials and sessions for individuals can be useful.

Group tutorials
Small groups of learners following a similar course may wish to come together as part of a self help programme. However, the learners may request the presence of a teacher from time to time to conduct a fairly formal tutorial around a given subject. Alternatively, you may wish to facilitate a series of group tutorials by setting up a timetable of sessions.

> *Six of my staff were following the Open University 'Nursing process' package. Once a week we got together to discuss some of the key subject areas. It was useful to make sure we were all talking about the same thing and to iron out any problems. We were able to reflect on our ideas, exchange information and follow up references. Each week we chose a different subject for the following week (eg evaluation). I would then prepare a short talk for the next week and we'd use that as the basis for the session. After a while, the staff started taking on board a topic each in turn themselves. Interestingly, this kept on going as a nursing process interest group long after the course had finished.*

Ward sister/clinical teacher

We found group tutorials very helpful, particularly as our staff are very scattered over a large unit, and some relatively isolated (eg by night duty). For many staff, getting back to learning was a new phenomenon and they seemed to find meeting other colleagues reinforcing to their studies, removing the 'I'm in this all alone and nobody understands' syndrome.

Personal tutorials

From time to time, most learners will feel the need for a tutorial session with a particular teacher. It may be that a regular programme of meetings is set up to cover specific topics, or they may be arranged on an ad-hoc basis as required by the learner. Sometimes the learner may simply need help with learning to learn again. Many students may not have undertaken any sort of formal learning for some time. Some open learning packages (for example Continuing Nurse Education Programme 1986) are also available to help with this. The important point seems to be that the learner has the option of such tutorials, as well as feeling comfortable about asking for them.

> *I have an 'open door' policy anyway as far as I'm concerned, with my office. I made it quite clear to Janet that she could come back to me if she got stuck anywhere in the programme. We had two or three particular occasions when we had to work quite hard at some subjects, but I think it helped her to get beyond them, then she was OK for a while and would come back to me if needs be.*

Nurse Tutor – conducting post-basic ENB courses

One thing that seems to be crucial is the tutor's 'style' or approach-ability in facilitating tutorials. Wong's (1979) study of fourteen students illustrated teacher behaviours which the students reported as helpful to their learning:

- demonstrating willingness to answer questions and offer explanations
- being interested in students and respectful to them
- giving students encouragement and due praise
- informing students of their progress
- displaying an appropriate sense of humour
- having a pleasant voice
- being available to students when needed
- giving an appropriate amount of supervision
- displaying confidence in themselves and in the students.

Teacher behaviours reported as being hindering to students' learning as identified by the students were:

- posing a threat
- being sarcastic
- acting in a superior manner
- belittling students
- correcting students in the presence of others
- supervising students too closely
- laying emphasis only on correcting the student's mistakes or pointing out their weakness.

Thus the teacher has to act as the knowledgeable resource person, acting as a facilitator, and with some very positive personal attributes if learning is going to be effective.

It may be that the teacher develops the personal tutorship further by setting up learning contracts with learners (Knowles 1984; Keyser 1986). The contract might be tied to a particular open learning package, or it may be part of a wider educational process of which the open learning unit is but one part. Knowles (1984) identifies the eight key elements, from the learners' point of view of a learning contract:

- diagnosing learning needs
- specifying the learning objectives
- specifying the learning resources and strategies needed
- specifying the evidence of accomplishment you can supply
- saying how the evidence will be evaluated
- reviewing the contract with peers, facilitators, etc.
- carrying out the contract
- evaluating learning.

The teacher has a key role in supporting the learner through this problem solving process. A full discussion of contract learning is beyond the scope of this text, but it is worth noting at this stage that

learning contracts can be a further useful educational tool in the open
learning process.

Acting as a personal tutor can provide essential additional support to
the learner in open learning. Offering choices, being a resource
person, sharing knowledge – are all essential contributions to helping
the learners in their chosen direction.

Personal counselling

This needs to be seen as quite separate and distinct from being a
personal tutor organising tutorials, and it is true that being trained as a
teacher does not guarantee that the person is also a trained counsellor.
The two sets of skills are quite distinct although they may have many
principles in common. Burnard (1985), Brandes and Ginnis (1986)
and Egan (1986) offer models of the counselling role of the teacher in
order to become a 'skilled helper'. It may well be that as a facilitator
for open learning, the teacher must also develop counselling skills and
learn to differentiate and adapt to these very different functions (this
issue is also discussed in Chapter 9).

Informal networks and self-help groups

These can be set up to provide a peer group support. It might mean,
for example, that a group of people undertaking a similar programme
of study are aware of each others addresses and telephone numbers.
Contact with a group or on a one to one basis can help clarify the
learners' ideas, seek advice or give assistance in the course. Networks
might be helpful locally, amongst peers and fellow learners, or can be
built up over a period of time over a wide range of colleagues to offer
mutual support. Sometimes these can be formalised into support
groups or self-help groups.

The teacher can help by participating in the network if required, and
facilitating self-help groups to get together eg by providing a room to
meet. Self-help groups can draw on the resources of others (for
example, inviting guest teachers to carry out tutorials or seminars) and
have the added advantage of combining the resources of this group.

> *We got together as a group and worked out a programme
> lasting over three months. The teachers let us have a
> classroom in the evening. On a couple of occasions, we
> clubbed together to organise and pay for speaker's expenses
> – we got one man to come in from the Parkinson's Disease
> Society, and another came from the Alzheimer's Society.*
>
> Ward Sister

The group is better equipped to share the cost of a journals club, for example, to pool information that is discovered, and to pass round copies of articles, share books and so on. It may in addition participate in fund raising to enhance the overall learning activities of a particular unit if this is appropriate (see above 'resources'). Sharing ideas, difficulties and successes can provide the support that is needed, especially if the course of study hits a difficult period, or help to remove the possibility of the learner feeling isolated from mainstream learning.

Although there are dangers of some individuals manipulating the purpose of the group, in the end the learners will determine the need for the group, select themselves into or out of it according to need, and the group can continue to exist for as long or as short a term as they feel necessary. The teacher can participate at their request, may help to clarify difficult issues or assist with difficult group dynamics. Self-help learning groups, by their very nature, tend to be transient, coming together to meet the needs of a particular group of people at a particular time and dispersing as the goals of the group have been met. It is also worth noting that group sessions and self-help groups formed part of an overall strategy for change on my unit. My colleagues and I wanted to avoid a 'top down' approach; we preferred a 'bottom up' approach where staff would take charge of their own learning and, by extension, of their own innovations in practice.

Supporting the learners in open and distance learning may be seen as a key role for the teachers. Both learners and teachers can derive enjoyment and stimulation from it. Acting as a resource and ideas person, a giver of options, a clarifier of ideas, a compass for direction and as a mirror for reflection, the teacher helps to empower the learners to take charge of their own learning.

References

Brandes G, Ginnis P 1986 *A Guide to Student Centred Learning.* Blackwell

Burnard P 1985 *Learning Human Skills, a guide for nurses.* Heinemann

Burns R 1982 *Self-concept Development and Education.* Holt, New York

Continuing Nurse Education Programme 1986 *Management of Learning – open learning for nurses.* Barnet College

Dickoff P, James J 1985 Theoretical pluralism. *A Direction for a Practice Discipline.* Ryerson School of Nursing, Toronto

Egan P 1986 *The Skilled Helper.* Brooks Cole

Ernst S, Goodison L 1981 *In Our Hands: a book of self help therapy*. Women's Press

English National Board 1987 *Managing Change in Nursing Education*. English National Board for Nursing, Midwifery and Health Visiting

Freire P 1973 *Education: The Practice of Freedom*. Writers and Readers Publishing Cooperative

Goffman I 1961 *Asylums*. Penguin

Goodall C J 1985 A student tutor's evaluation of his teaching placement. *Nurse Education Today*, 5

Hopson B, Scally M 1981 *Lifeskills Teaching*. McGraw Hill, New York

Hurst K 1985 Traditional versus progressive nurse education : a review of the literature. *Nurse Education Today*, 5, pp103-8

Knowles M 1984 *The Adult Learner, a neglected species*. Gulf Publishing, Houston

Ombudsman's Report 1986-8 *Report of the Health Commissioner*. Department of Health

Pearson A, Vaughan B 1986 *Nursing Models for Practice*. Heinemann

Price Waterhouse 1988 *Nurse Retention and Recruitment*. Price Waterhouse

Purdy E, Wright S G 1988 If I were a rich nurse. *Nursing Times* 84 (40) pp42-3

RCN 1986 *The Education of Nurses – a new dispensation*. Royal College of Nursing

Rogers C 1983 *Freedom to Learn for the 80's*. Merrill, New York

Royal Commission on the National Health Service 1979. HMSO

UKCC 1986 *Project 2000 – a new preparation for practice*. United Kingdom Central Council for Nursing, Midwifery and Health Visiting

Wong S 1979 Nurse-teacher behaviours in the clinical field: apparent effect on nursing students' learning. *Journal of Advanced Nursing* 3, pp369-78

Wright S G 1986 *Building and Using a Model of Nursing*. Arnold

11 The Diploma in Nursing: a study centre network

Kate Robinson

The Diploma in Nursing which is run by the Distance Learning Centre (DLC) was the first substantial national distance learning programme leading to a qualification to be established for nurses in the UK. The Diploma, which is validated by the University of London, is a 2-3 year part-time course; it is based mainly on the acquisition of academic knowledge but it also includes components based on the acquisition of practice competencies. It is run by a number of colleges of further and higher education which base their curriculum on the syllabus and regulations produced by the University. Although the DLC curriculum follows the syllabus and regulations of the University, unlike other courses offering the same qualification, ninety per cent of the course is taught 'at a distance' through the use of learning materials such as text and audio-tape produced by the DLC, and only ten per cent based on face to face tuition provided locally. It is this ten per cent, and particularly the organisation of it, which I want to examine here. In order to do that it will be useful to begin by reviewing briefly the original process of negotiation and validation which led to the existing framework.

Planning the local element

Because the course required validation by the University of London, the Extra-mural Department of the University, which administered the Diploma, was an early partner in the planning process (the extra-mural department has subsequently become part of Birkbeck College). In order to deal with a submission which was clearly seen as out of the ordinary, they convened a validation group to explore the problems and solutions *before* a formal request for validation was made.

A number of alternatives were discussed in vague terms but it was made clear that validation would not be forthcoming for a programme which relied entirely on distance learning materials and tuition at a distance from the DLC. This principle did not rest on any objection to distance learning as such but in the fact that a wholly distance based system would have violated one of the tenets of the course, namely that collaboration between an institution of further or higher education and the health authority which employs the students is essential for the success of the students in the work-based part of the curriculum. The notion of partnership was therefore central to the philosophy of the course. While a distance learning programme run from the DLC could easily support the academic side of the partnership, it had no health authority attachments to build on and it was not easy to see how a national educational centre could have appropriate links with a health authority. Clearly an acceptable proposal would link the DLC to each student *and* to their health authority, but the proposed student numbers ran into hundreds and possibly thousands; it was inconceivable that the DLC could enter into negotiations with each student's health authority separately.

Possible models

Although the Diploma was the first such scheme for nursing there were precedents within open learning of educational institutions which produced and distributed learning materials nationally and also offered students local support. The most obvious example was the Open University but there was also the Flexistudy programme of the NEC.

The Open University

The Open University operates a network of Regional Centres where a core team of academic and administrative staff, headed by a Regional Director, is based. The part-time tutorial staff and the students are also attached to one of these regional centres, although they may never actually go there because of the distance nature of the work. The examples of regional responsibilities given in the Student handbook (Open University 1987) include the maintenance of student records, the organisation of tutorial and counselling sessions, residential schools, day schools and examinations, and the building of contacts with local organisations such as local education authorities, libraries, etc.

The regional centres are entirely independent of any other local educational institution; they belong to the Open University. An analogy would be the French colonies which were legally part of mainland France despite their geographical separation. Each regional centre operates a network of small Study Centres based in other colleges. The study centres, of which there are about 250 throughout the UK (Open University 1987), may provide meeting rooms, a common room, library and refreshment facilities and opportunities for consulting academic and administrative Open University publications.

However, the separation of the Open University local support centres from other educational institutions does not correspond with the early plans:

> The early papers of the Advisory Committee and the Planning Committee envisaged co-operative academic work between the Open University and the WEA, the extra-mural departments of the universities and the Local Education Authorities. In practice such direct academic collaboration has developed, if at all, only very slowly.
>
> Perry 1976

There was collaboration, of course, but centred on the administrative arrangements for renting the facilities from the local college. The Open University, as Perry admits, is essentially parasitic upon the local institutions. Many of the staff of the local colleges have become part-time tutors for the Open University and have thus gained personally through teaching a different group of students and a wider range of courses, and such gains will indirectly affect the local college. But the potential of academic collaboration between the Open University and local colleges and other institutions envisaged in the early planning has never been taken up.

The National Extension College

The NEC staff both produce learning materials and tutor courses but the NEC also has a number of collaborative arrangements with local colleges, the most well known of which is called FlexiStudy. FlexiStudy (which is a trade mark) was developed by Barnet College in the early 1970s to offer a more flexible service to students who were not able to attend their conventional courses on a regular basis. Using the learning materials produced by the NEC they integrated them into a system of locally offered resources including tutorials, counselling by post and telephone and library access as in this account:

> Enrolment on a FlexiStudy course at a college of further, higher or adult education entitles a student to what is, in effect, a 'total learning package'. The college supplies complete NEC correspondence course materials plus the services of a staff tutor who marks written work and provides tutorial support by letter, telephone and in face-to-face seminars. Additionally, FlexiStudy students have access to all facilities normally open to college students – science and language laboratories for practical work,

library and audiovisual resources, careers and counselling services, examination entry, canteen, etc.

National Extension College 1979, cited in Jenkins and Perraton 1980

This system was developed by a college and remains controlled by the individual colleges which affiliate to it. They enrol their own students and offer tutorial support by their own staff who remain employed by the college, although their contracts may be changed to accommodate the necessity of flexibility.

The DLC study centre network

In addition to the advantages and disadvantages displayed by these models the DLC also had to consider the preferences of the University of London for substantial links between the institution running the course and the student's employers. The structure which was finally arrived at was a network of study centres which could deliver support to the student locally and provide a manageable link between the student and the DLC and the employer and the DLC. Ideally, such a network should have been established with a centre in each health authority so that access could be assured for any student regardless of their place of work. However, there were a number of reasons why this was not possible, and indeed has not yet been achieved. Firstly, negotiating with well over 200 health authorities simultaneously was not within the capacity of the DLC. Secondly, the concept of a study centre within the Diploma network involves a positive commitment from the local health authority management and many Regions and Districts were uninterested in augmenting their existing provision. The health authority does not just 'host' the centre on a contractual basis as is the case with Open University study centres, they are *part of* the study centre.

What is a study centre?

The most important characteristic of the DLC study centre is that it is not a place or a building but '...a network of resources which will support the students locally while they undertake the distance learning course.' (South Bank Polytechnic 1986). The students need access to some physical resources such as libraries and, because of the vocational nature of the course, they also need support in their clinical areas. The organisation of a study centre is undertaken by a consortium of interested parties which must include representation from clinical and educational sectors either from one health authority or from a group of health authorities and educational institutions, although it is assumed that all the employers of the students on the course will normally be represented. Usually this consortium is part of an existing post-registration education liaison committee in some form and the arrangements for the Diploma becomes part of a network of collaborating arrangements.

The guidelines for the necessary resources and the composition of the consortium were part of the DLC submission to the University of London and thereafter the approval of each individual centre can be done by the DLC. This ensures that the network of study centres can grow in response to local needs without any lengthy and complicated resubmission procedures.

The distribution of proposed resource input within a consortium can be summarised as follows:

- the DLC was to provide the teaching materials, which contain the whole of the syllabus, the assessment of assignments, and a tutor-counsellor to provide tuition and counselling locally;
- the local teaching institution(s) were to provide the facilities, such as seminar rooms, audio-visual equipment and the library;
- the employing institution was to provide, for the majority of the students, the time and financial resources to undertake the programme, and the facilities for the workplace learning element and the workplace mentors.

Tutor-counsellors

The students were to receive their local support from a tutor-counsellor attached to the study centre. She would probably be employed as a tutor by one of the institutions involved in the consortium but for the purposes of supporting the Diploma students she was to be employed by the DLC on a part-time basis. This could be arranged on a secondment basis with the contract being between the DLC and her employer but it did allow the DLC to take a direct interest in the quality of the support to be provided to the students. According to the submission document (South Bank Polytechnic 1986) the duties of the tutor-counsellor were to:

- offer regular tuition and counselling to their students both individually and in groups
- liaise as necessary with the students' employers
- advise students on any financial arrangements or help that might be available locally
- assist in the evaluation of the course
- recruit and brief the facilitator network and maintain good liaison with it

- keep adequate records
- liaise between the DLC and the study centre and advise the DLC on any problems or inadequacy in local resources.

This last duty shows the importance of the tutor-counsellor having strong links with the DLC as well as to their main employer. A number of the listed duties are radically different from those of tutor-counsellors within the Open University system and reflect the vocational nature of the Diploma course. The tutor-counsellor's local knowledge would be essential for, for example, recruiting facilitators who have a commitment to professional development and an up-to-date knowledge of nursing developments. And unlike Open University tutor-counsellors they were required to offer face-to-face individual tuition to each student as well as group work.

Again unlike Open University tutor-counsellors, they were not required to mark the students' assignments, which were to be marked centrally at the DLC. This was the subject of some controversy, as not all the validating committee were happy with splitting the counselling function from the assessment function both on pedagogic and logistical grounds. Pedagogically it was thought that the tutor-counsellors should be involved with all aspects of the students' activities and that formal assessment should be integrated into the learning process. The counter argument was that within the existing Diploma structures where marking was carried out by an internal assessor, an external assessor and a chief assessor, the assessment process was already separated out to some extent. Furthermore, each student would only have one tutor-counsellor who would be most unlikely to be able to mark all the topic areas covered by the assignments in three years of study. The logistical argument concerned the difficulty of feeding back comments on the students' problems in time for them to be discussed before the next assignment. This was solved in part by producing feedback forms, which would include advice but no grade, which were to be completed by the internal assessor and sent back to the students at the time of internal marking and before the final grade had been agreed. However, the separation of face-to-face tuition and counselling from formal assessment was seen as an interim solution which might require amendment, particularly if the tutor-counsellors wished to be involved with the formal assessment of the course.

The Diploma course can be characterised as distance rather than open learning (for a discussion of distance and open learning *see* Chapter 2) and the role of the tutor-counsellor was not therefore necessarily designed to be as involved with some aspects of student self-reflection and personal growth as with an more 'open' course, although of course the possibility for such work is always there. Her role was seen primarily as promoting independent study skills and supporting the academic content of the course. The latter poses particular problems as the content of the course syllabus is so broad. The tutor-counsellors were therefore to be supported in turn by unit coordinators, that is those academics who were coordinating the production of a unit of the Diploma course (which consists of six units, two being studied each year). It was assumed that most problems would occur in the first year of course presentation when defects in the materials would come to light and questions be directed at the tutor-counsellors; in subsequent years the unit coordinators could brief tutor-counsellors about likely problems. Although the tutor-counsellors were only to be given one briefing session a year, communication by post and telephone could be more extensive. The tutor-counsellors were to be consulted individually about the problems of the course and the students, but they also had a representative on the Course Board.

Evaluation

The scheme was validated by the University in 1986 and has since had two student intakes. It is therefore possible to begin to evaluate the structures which were established and to ask whether any issues or problems were overlooked or indeed whether the DLC structure offers particular advantages over the other models of support for students on a vocational course. First it might be helpful to review the two non-vocational models from the Open University and the NEC.

The systems compared

These two systems, the Open University regional network and the local confederation of colleges offering FlexiStudy, are very different. First, they are not comparable in size as the Open University system provides national coverage and caters for many more students on a long term basis. Second, they differ in the important elements of ownership of support staff and students. However, both seem to offer the students involved a satisfactory service within the aims they have established for themselves. Nevertheless, from the point of view of the central institution it could be argued that the ownership is important. Certainly it enables:

- closer quality control of student support
- consistency of support
- a more complete institutional profile.

All these factors were particularly important when the Open University was established in 1969. Although it has subsequently achieved an enormous success, gaining national and international recognition, it must be remembered that at its foundation failure was being widely predicted. It therefore seemed necessary to establish the Open University as a 'complete' institution which could offer all the services which a conventional university would supply, and to a comparable standard. Mike Richardson, in comparing the two institutions comments:

> It seems on balance likely that NEC has suffered for the lack of a regional structure of its own. Yet it has been spared the not insignificant expense of such an operation and has perhaps been led more directly towards local collaboration in one of its most successful forms, namely FlexiStudy. Nonetheless, it has been the quality of the support services available to students through the regional structure which has, in large measure, distinguished the Open University from comparable institutions overseas and has been a significant factor in securing the high level of student survival and progress.
>
> Richardson 1988

However, although the regional structure has clearly benefited the Open University, from the point of view of the educational system as a whole and the host institutions in particular, the boundaries imposed by the Open University may be considered to have inhibited their development. If the institutions had been more involved in the Open University, they might have benefited from contact with Open University students who are mature students, more of their staff could have had the opportunity for some work at a more advanced level, and the ideas of open access and distance teaching, which have only recently infiltrated the further and higher education sectors could have gained ground much sooner.

A summary of the important issues in student support systems would therefore include the following:

- establishing an national independent support structure is very costly and time consuming
- the quality of the support service is vital to the reputation of the central institution as well as to student success
- collaboration with existing local teachers and others could promote the ideas of open learning within the institutions.

How does the DLC network compare?
The initial cohort of students on the Diploma in Nursing were attached to nine study centres scattered throughout the UK and extending from Jersey to Inverness. Since then one centre has stopped recruiting students, although the existing cohort will continue, and others have

joined. The goal of national coverage is still far from achieved, however, and this presents difficulties to students who move during the course. From this point of view any network which depends on individual initiatives by each local centre will necessarily be incomplete, and of course the process of individual negotiation will be time-consuming. It is a system which gives power to the employer, to opt in or out, but not to the individual employee who might want to use such a service.

Quality control has not been a major issue although there has been some renegotiation between the DLC and the tutor-counsellors about their duties, for example, tutors are now much more involved in recruitment. The success of students depends on a number of factors other than academic capability, and the tutor-counsellor is best placed to know when work and sometimes personal commitments would impede a student's progress. With regard to the use of materials it has become apparent that the tutor-counsellor often has to adapt the materials to local conditions. Within Unit 4, for example, it has proved extremely difficult to produce materials which deal with equal thoroughness with nursing organisational structures throughout the UK. At times the authors have suggested that subjects are best dealt with by the tutor-counsellors within the group work sessions. So although the group work sessions were intended to be entirely at the discretion of the local tutor-counsellor and students some fairly heavy hints have been given. This is, of course, a two way process as the tutor-counsellors have also made suggestions to the authors about how the materials should be changed.

There are indications that the tutor-counsellors are devoting more time to their Diploma work than is specified in the contract. This is partly because in the first year of the course the tutor-counsellors have to read all the materials for the first time, in effect they have to study the course with the students, but also because they feel that many students need a lot of help to cope with the demands of the course. This tension between offering the learner more independence and the desire to give more student support is a common one in open learning and is frequently debated within the Open University where students press for more tutorials. It could be argued that the freedom granted by open learning is the freedom to fail, but it may be unreasonable to expect nurses, many of whom who were trained in a rigid didactic educational system, to cope with the demands of open learning overnight. This problem may be exacerbated by the small numbers of students studying at some centres; group cohesion and peer support may overcome many of the problems of open learning, but groups of three or four may have insufficient internal resources. The demands made on the support staff where open learning is recently introduced and introduced on a small scale may therefore be excessive. And, of course, like the students the tutor-counsellors had to fit this new role into existing roles and duties and conflicts did occur. Some centres have acknowledged that extra resources are required and have invested the resources of the part-time post of tutor-counsellor into the partial funding of a team of tutors who support the students and each other. In this case the institution rather than the individual tutor is adding additional resources to the support facilities.

The Diploma was established as a full cost course and, from the point of view of the DLC, a central problem was the cost-effectiveness of each individual tutor-counsellor. A payment model had been adapted from the Open University whereby the tutor-counsellor (or her employer) was paid a flat fee plus an additional fee related to the numbers of students. Obviously if just one student enrolled the tutor-counsellor fee was still substantial although the income from the student was negligible. This was a particular problem in the first year of presentation before student numbers built up through the accumulation of yearly cohorts. The problem has been partially solved by the imposition of minimal student quotas but this really only ameliorates the problem. It is essentially a characteristic of full cost courses, the economics of which must be based on the costs of a group. Within open learning the problem is exacerbated because the system depends on the economies of scale, which can be lost if the costs are not evenly distributed, as is almost inevitable in any system of local study centres. The Open University solves this problem to some extent by making the recruitment of tutors dependent on student registrations. However, if tutor-counsellors are needed to provide a continuous service, and if they are an integral part of the consortium, as in the DLC, then this option is not available. One solution is the input of resource from the local employer to compensate for when the local group is too small to be economic.

A central question must be the relationship of the support network with the central academic unit. This relationship has been problematic within the Open University (Perry 1976) which has changed its structures to deal with the problem. Although the DLC initially envisaged each study centre as an individual entity with a direct one-to-one relationship with the DLC, the creation of a tutor-counsellor support group has changed this perception. Within a month of the start of the course the tutor-counsellors, who had met at the pre-course briefing meeting, had formed the support group which could then begin to deal directly with the DLC (Robinson 1988). It is probably the case that the DLC depends on its tutor-counsellors rather more than the Open University does, not only for the support which they give the students but for the support which they give the DLC within the consortium. The consortium contains the employers whose financial support of the students makes the course possible, and an adverse report by the tutor-counsellor could change the level of future support. However, this power does not extend to academic issues, the tutor-counsellors cannot, for example, respond to the needs of their students by negotiating changes in the curriculum because those matters are determined by the University of London.

A main theme of this discussion has been that the distance learning model Diploma in Nursing run by the Distance Learning Centre operates within a complex structure incorporating the University of London, the DLC, which is part of South Bank Polytechnic, and a network of study centres throughout the UK. The system owes something to the structures of the Open University but it has unique features which meet the particular needs of the students of the DLC and the requirements of the University of London. However, the final form of the structure was not arrived at without a great deal of discussion and debate, which only rarely became acrimonious, and the history of that process illustrates a number of the issues pertaining to the support of students within a formal assessed open learning system. The issues involved in the establishment of support networks for students on formal open learning courses are likely to become increasingly important with the establishment of open learning in the health service. For example, the National Health Service Training Authority MESOL programme (Management Education Syllabus and Open Learning project), which may be assessed by either the Open University or the Institute of Health Services Management, has a system of tutors and mentors. And as nursing courses similarly turn to open learning as a major route for post-registration education the nursing profession may have to make important decisions about the nature and control of the support system or systems. Analysis of the existing models may form a helpful part of that debate.

References

Jenkins J and Perraton H 1980 *The Invisible College NEC 1963-1979*. IEC Broadsheets on Distance Learning No 15, International Extension College

Perry W 1976 *Open University* The Open University Press

Richardson M 1988 The National Extension College and the Open University – a comparison of two national institutions. In Paine N (ed.) *Open Learning in Transition*. National Extension College

Robinson K M 1988 The distance learning mode diploma in nursing: a case study of collaboration *International Journal of Nursing Studies* 25, 4, pp271-7

South Bank Polytechnic 1986 *Course submission document: part-time Diploma in Nursing*. Distance Learning Centre

12 Hybrid courses in continuing professional development

Elisabeth Clark

The fundamental importance of continuing education has been demonstrated in a number of studies (Lathlean 1986; Rogers and Lawrence 1987), but concern has also been expressed about the barriers restricting nurses' access to the opportunities available (Farnish 1983). Within continuing education generally, the importance and benefits of a well educated workforce are increasingly acknowledged, and many educators and trainers have been involved in discussions about how to 'transmit' knowledge and skills effectively to a wide and varied population of adult learners who comprise a very heterogeneous group. Indeed this whole issue has become even more important in the light of changing demographic patterns, difficulties in retaining qualified staff, and a general reduction in levels of funding at a time when the costs of providing conventional education and training courses continue to escalate. Given this background, it is clear that traditional approaches to education are not going to satisfy the demands of the future. It has, therefore, become all the more urgent to examine the possible contribution of open learning. For open learning, by its very nature, can provide solutions, as will be seen, to the problems of providing learning experiences for registered nurses.

Prior to the 1960s, relatively little was known about the characteristics of adult learning; much of the research in education had been concerned with the teaching and learning of children and young people. However, it is now well understood that adults learn – and therefore need to be taught – in ways that differ considerably from those that apply to children in school. Knowles (1987), for example, lists several characteristics of adult learning that need to be acknowledged if continuing education programmes are to be effective. He argues that adults on the one hand have a deep psychological need to be self-directing, but on the other hand have usually been conditioned by previous educational experiences to be dependent and to think of education as 'being taught'. So much so that many people initially feel uncomfortable about being given responsibility for their own learning. Consequently, many adult learners will need help to become less dependent and to accept greater responsibility for their own learning. It is also evident that adult learners bring with them a wealth of life experiences and a wide range of individual needs. It is therefore essential that all continuing professional education programmes should be designed with a high degree of flexibility.

Open learning aims to create new opportunities for learning by removing many of the barriers and constraints associated with conventional education and training schemes. Compared with college attendance at set times and traditional teaching techniques such as lectures, its flexible, learner-centred, interactive approach to education and training is widely recognised (Dixon 1987). Open learning would, therefore, appear to be particularly well suited to meeting the specific needs of adult learners wishing to study while remaining in the workforce. Courses are increasingly likely to be offered in modular form so that students can select specific modules relevant to their particular interests and needs, and build up a programme of learning to meet their own circumstances and career aspirations. Pragmatically, it is a very useful way of extending the range of a syllabus when a course is dependent on a small pool of teaching staff who may have neither the time nor the subject expertise to increase the numbers of modules offered. However, the successful application of open learning to continuing professional education requires that its advantages be fully understood and effectively exploited. In particular, the possibilities, benefits and practical implications of incorporating open learning materials into a teaching programme need to be considered.

The hybrid model

Many people tend to think in terms of mutually exclusive alternatives – either face-to-face teaching *or* open learning – with the former being the preferred alternative. However, it is well known that open learning materials are being used within conventional courses in a number of ways, both overt and covert (Stainton Rogers 1983). Lawrence *et al* (1988) confirm that this is also true in nursing: 'The majority of the distance learning materials used by districts in the sample have been used as part of existing courses or to provide a core for a new but still "taught" course.' Stainton Rogers has proposed a number of models for what she calls 'the alternative use of materials' (Stainton Rogers 1987), a phrase which she further defines as '...any situation where one person or a group of people make use of learning materials (text, videotape, audiotape, etc.) produced by other people, for a teaching purpose other than that for which they were originally designed'. She suggests that materials producers could plan their production knowing that such alternative use was likely, and render the materials more flexible and adaptable.

In this chapter I want to describe one instance of the use of materials which were produced in just this way: the Research Awareness programme produced by the Distance Learning Centre. The course team planning the materials intended that, as a minimum, they could be used for Unit 5 of the Diploma in Nursing (University of London) syllabus, ENB 995 *An Introduction to the Understanding and Application of Research* (now ENB 870), and as a series of free standing modules to be used by individual learners or incorporated into a variety of in-service post-registration educational opportunities. I will be describing a course which consists of part face-to-face teaching and part independent learning based on open learning materials, and I shall use the term 'hybrid' because I want to argue that, like hybrid plants, such courses have increased vigour! It has always been acknowledged that a lot of useful learning occurs outside the classroom, lecture theatre or laboratory. The importance of private study, further reading, small group discussions and so on, all testify to this. Moreover, the Council for National Academic Awards (CNAA) will now give academic credit to knowledge and competence acquired in the workplace if it can be assessed. Yet despite this recognition, the majority of continuing education courses continue to place considerable emphasis on face-to-face teaching. In this context, any self-directing component seems to take second place, either as a means of reinforcing what has been learned in the classroom, or, for the more able student, as a means of supplementing their learning.

Both open learning and face-to-face teaching have advantages and disadvantages. Cropley and Kahl (1983) have identified a number of characteristics associated with each. Face-to-face teaching is characterised by more immediate personal contact between learner and teacher; the teacher is more directly in control of learning although the learners may experience a limited degree of freedom; a high degree of feedback and therefore evaluation by the teacher is possible. In this situation, a learner's internal motivation, self-direction, ability and willingness to work without direct supervision may be low.

In contrast, there is less personal contact in open learning; the teacher's influence tends to be indirect; learners experience a greater degree of freedom; less external feedback and evaluation is usually possible. In such circumstances, the learner's commitment, internal motivation, self-direction and willingness and ability to work without direct supervision need to be high.

Whilst recognising that any attempt to characterise different modes of teaching inevitably leads to gross over-simplification, each of the two situations described has its positive and negative side. Consequently I would like to propose that, by careful mixing of the two modes in a particular educational context, it is possible to retain many of the advantages, whilst avoiding some of the disadvantages, of each.

The benefits of hybridisation

From the learner's point of view, the use of combined face-to-face and open learning modes provide greater flexibility and improved access for those who are unable, because of work or personal commitments, to attend a course requiring regular attendance at set times in a particular location. Moreover, a combined course might well attract both learners who dislike formal teaching-learning situations and also those who would not contemplate enrolling for a course taught purely at a distance. The contact with and support of the teachers and other group members has been found to reduce the isolation felt by some learners in learning at a distance. And if a problem should arise when studying alone, it is almost certainly easier to contact by letter or telephone someone with whom you have had personal contact during the face-to-face component of the course.

Mixed mode courses can also bring benefits to the providers of education, whether they be the employing agency or an institute of higher education. Whenever face-to-face teaching is the central component of any course, this inevitably limits the number of students who can be involved at any one time and, therefore constrains access. Planned use of self-directed learning using open learning materials within an overall educational programme can facilitate the education of larger numbers of learners in a way that might not be feasible or cost effective if face-to-face teaching alone were used. Such courses can be both educationally successful and economically viable. Moreover, the reduction in the number of class contact hours releases accommodation, which is often at a premium in many institutions of higher education and health authorities, and frees staff time, enabling more courses to be run or making available time for important non-teaching activities such as staff development. Moreover, as Stainton Rogers (1987) argues:

> There are good reasons for deciding to incorporate materials produced by somebody else into your own teaching. Very often such materials will have been produced by an organisation with access to skilled staff, and considerable resources in terms of the facilities and equipment for the generation of high quality text, video and audiotape... considerable time and effort has already been expended in their development.

Clearly the financial costs and benefits of incorporating open learning materials into a course need to be examined. On the one hand, there is the cost of buying the material in the first place, and of replacing it if students are allowed to retain the materials after the course has ended. Against this, one has to remember the real costs of providing face-to-face tuition. If one includes the cost of teacher's time or fees, administration, replacement staff, plus subsidies for student travel and subsistence then the real price is high.

The constraints

But before assuming that mixed mode courses offer the ideal solution it is important to stress a number of points. First, within the overall course programme any open learning component needs to be properly integrated into the overall course philosophy and curriculum, and planned from the start. Any differences in the underlying principles of different components in a mixed mode course would readily be apparent to students. It would, for instance, be very confusing to students to try to combine a highly teacher centred and teacher controlled taught component guided by prescriptive behavioural objectives with flexible open learning materials which had been designed to encourage individual students to identify and meet their own learning needs. In short, a prerequisite of any course is that it should be based on a coherent educational philosophy and a consistent set of teaching principles, irrespective of the mode of presentation of any particular part of the programme. Tutors need, therefore, to be entirely familiar with the open learning materials if they are to be effectively linked to other teaching inputs.

Needless to say, the use of open learning materials does not imply a diminished role for the course teachers but a changed role. Traditionally the teacher is seen as subject expert with responsibility for teaching, motivating, assessing, counselling and supporting students and monitoring their progress. Whilst many of these activities continue to be important, the key role of the teacher is no longer that of information transmitter when open learning materials are being used, but rather that of facilitator; the need to stimulate and support students becomes their most crucial function (Paley 1986, Thorpe 1988). This arises from a fundamental change in educational philosophy, including a commitment to hand over a considerable amount of responsibility and control of learning to the individual student. Overall, this represents a significant shift of emphasis from teaching to learning, encouraging individuals to take greater responsibility for their own learning, and helping to produce the new type of practitioner envisaged by Project 2000. Although the idea of using open learning materials may initially seem threatening to many teachers who feel they have become redundant in this process, it is important to remember that the concept of self-directed learning is crucial to effective adult learning.

As facilitators of learning, teachers encourage students to help themselves. Overall, this represents a significant shift of emphasis from teaching to learning and involves encouraging individuals to take greater responsibility for their own learning, and supporting them in this endeavour. By combining opportunities for self-directed learning with face-to-face teaching a more student oriented rather than teacher oriented programme can be achieved. It should, however, be noted in passing, that the term 'independent learner' or 'independent learning' can imply a number of different things (Morgan 1985). On the positive side, as we have already seen, it can describe students taking responsibility for what and how they study and developing greater self-direction in learning. It is also used to refer to the physical separation between teacher and learner and as such is a basic ingredient of any open learning course. Unfortunately, it can also be used to justify cutting back on the overall amount of tuition and support available for students.

Finally, the learning materials used for the self-directed component of any course must be of high academic quality. Originally some concern was expressed about whether open learning courses could achieve the same standards as equivalent conventionally taught courses (Perry 1976). However, the high standards set by the Open University have helped to dispel many anxieties. More recently, the publication entitled *Ensuring Quality in Open Learning: A handbook for action* (Manpower Services Commission 1988) should also make a significant contribution to the maintenance of standards, as many different groups and organisations became involved in producing and using open learning materials. Its Code of Practice represents the accumulated experience of a number of experts in open learning and must be viewed as an important step in the process of establishing national standards of quality in open learning. The handbook stresses from the outset the fact that 'quality in open learning – from market research through to design, production, dissemination and support services – never arises automatically, just by accident or good fortune'. Quality needs to be planned and built into all open learning systems. A similar message is conveyed by the ENB *Criteria for approval of courses with an open learning component.*

Good open learning materials will stimulate students' interest and involvement, and can facilitate the transfer of learning from classroom to the workplace. They will provide a framework within which individual students or small groups can acquire knowledge and think through theoretical issues for themselves and relate these to their own experience. The key to effective learning at a distance is the interactive nature of the materials. By this I mean that the text does not merely give learners information but involves them in using the material. For instance, activities requiring a personal response from the student are a central part of the learning experience and encourage students to take greater responsibility for their own learning. This involvement can take a number of different forms, such as answering questions, seeking the opinions of others (such as colleagues and patients), finding out specific information about one's local area, carrying out particular activities and evaluating the outcome. Through the use of activities, open learning materials offer an effective means of helping students to relate theory to practice and, surprisingly to some, they can offer a very effective means of changing attitudes (Stainton Rogers 1986).

There are likely to be numerous reasons why teachers decide to incorporate open learning materials into their own teaching programmes. It may be that the necessary expertise is lacking locally, or that a teacher wishes to experiment with using different forms of teaching and learning. Alternatively, they may be used because of their flexibility or as a means of helping adult students to accept greater responsibility for their learning and encouraging self-directed learning. Whatever the reason, the use of open learning materials should never be viewed as an 'easy option'. We have already considered some of the benefits and constraints; a case study of one mixed mode course will enable us to examine some of the logistics and detail of introducing such a course.

A case study

I shall take as my example a course which I helped to plan and set up that was validated by the English National Board (ENB) and run at Essex Institute of Higher Education (now part of Anglia Higher Education College): ENB 995:*An Introduction to the Understanding and Application of Research* (now ENB 870).

The pilot course was run in 1985-6 and a mixed mode course has been offered every year since then. This thirty-day course was designed to include eleven days of self-directed learning based on open learning materials; the remaining nineteen days were College based, involving lectures, seminars, group discussions and tutorials. For the self-directed learning component of the course, students worked at their own pace through seven modules selected from the thirteen modules of the Research Awareness programme produced by the Distance Learning Centre (DLC), South Bank Polytechnic. Although these materials provided students with some direction, they also offered a degree of freedom about how they chose to approach their learning. Whilst their learning was not truly self-directed in the Rogerian sense, the use of open learning materials can act as a means of acquiring self-directing learning skills.

For a hybrid course, the teachers need to decide which parts of the curriculum are to be taught using specific open learning modules. This decision is usually made on a pragmatic basis according to what materials are available and their appropriateness to the overall course philosophy. As author of many of the modules, and closely involved in the production of the remaining ones, familiarity with the materials was not a problem. However, when planning to incorporate open learning materials into any course, it is obviously necessary for teachers to be totally familiar with the principles, structure and organisation of those materials, in much the same way that the Open University expects its tutors to familiarise themselves with the materials for the courses they teach. This highlights the desirability for there to be an ongoing dialogue between producers of open learning materials and consumers. Many useful ideas and practical tips could be exchanged. In this instance, each of the modules in the Research Awareness programme is intended to complement the other modules, but has also been designed to be free-standing or self-contained. Hence each identifies at the outset what key concepts need to be understood before embarking on that particular module. This flexibility is intended to facilitate the use of any module or selection of modules as part of conventionally taught courses.

The overall aims are stated clearly at the beginning of every module as follows:

- to promote professional self-awareness
- to encourage all nurses, midwives and health visitors to develop a questioning approach to their work
- to extend knowledge about research and its application to professional practice
- to encourage cross-fertilisation of ideas between practitioners and researchers, based on mutual respect and collaboration.

The materials are not highly prescriptive nor are they based on teacher-oriented objectives. This philosophy is reflected in a number of ways. The scene for each module is set by a short descriptive section entitled 'About this module', rather than a list of behavioural objectives. The activities are designed to help students, whether working individually or in small groups, to explore issues raised in the text and relate them directly to their own work situation. Each activity is followed by a commentary which discusses the main points raised by that particular activity. Often there will not be a single 'correct' answer to an activity, so many of the commentaries encourage students to look at their own responses in the light of the comments made (*see* Figure 12.1).

Furthermore, the final activity of each module asks individual students to identify and reflect on what they have learned, since it is assumed that this will in part be determined by their own particular background, current interests and specific needs. The final activity also encourages students to consider how they intend to use this knowledge in their day-to-day work (*see* Figure 12.2).

G

Activity 2.4   *Allow 5 minutes*

Below are listed six different kinds of authority that you are likely to refer
to. Identify which of these you use, and for each of those provide a specific
example of who/what you consulted and describe your reason(s) for
consulting that particular authority.

Written authority

- text book
- procedure or policy document
- journal.

People who can be an authority

- nurse manager
- specialist nurse
- medical consultant.

Commentary

*When you have completed this exercise, you might like to think about
any other people to whom you go for advice, and whether you are
obliged to follow the advice that you are given. You should also
consider who has the power to control your nursing practice. Advice
and authority can be vested in different people, in which case a conflict
may arise. This raises the interesting question of how far the
responsibility rests with the individual nurse to make decisions for
herself.*

Figure 12.1 Encouraging students to look at their own responses

Integrating the components

However, once this decision is made, the open learning components
need to be embedded within the overall course structure as in the
following example related to the teaching of a research method.
Module 9 *The Experimental Perspective* (DLC 1988) was used as the
core teaching material for that part of the course connected with
experimental research. Immediately prior to the one and a half days
set aside in the programme to work through the module, students were
given a face-to-face session in which key issues were identified to help
them orient themselves to the materials. In addition, the experimental
method was placed in a wider discussion concerning different research
methods and their related assumptions. The start of the next college
based day was also set aside for any exchange of ideas, discussion and
follow-up that was needed. During these sessions it became apparent
that it was important to allow the students themselves to use this time
as they pleased. There is a real danger that such sessions become a
teacher-led means of checking that key concepts have been
understood – thus focusing perhaps on the anxieties of the tutor

---

Final Activity *However long it takes*

Think back over this module and write down the major points that you have learned from it. When you have completed this, note down any specific ways in which you intend to use this knowledge in your work situation.

Commentary
Can you now identify three major sources of nursing knowledge with increased confidence and discuss their relative merits? You should also be able to discuss the contribution of common sense to nursing knowledge. I hope that this module will encourage you to recognise the sources of your own nursing knowledge and evaluate their appropriateness, and also to question the basis of authority, including clinical nursing policy and procedure documents that you regularly use. In your turn you should also try to encourage colleagues to do some of the activities that you have found particularly useful. Only when the majority of nurses are aware of the basis of their knowledge and begin to question their practice will the urgent need for reliable information on which to base decisions be recognised by the nursing profession at large.

Figure 12.2 Encouraging students to consider how to use their own knowledge in their day-to-day work

rather than those of the students, and at the same time taking away from the students some of the responsibility for their own learning. It soon became obvious that, thanks to the use of the end of section 'progress boxes' which provide a brief summary of the main points covered, and the self-assessment questions with answers given at the end of the module, students were able to check their own understanding. If further revision was needed then this would be raised and dealt with by the group, and could usually be resolved by peer teaching.

After the follow-up sessions, the students then received some additional teaching about the use of statistics and the analysis of data since this was not considered by the course teachers to have been covered in sufficient depth in the module. Also, it was the experience of the teachers that students frequently need to have their self-confidence boosted in any matter relating to numerical analysis. Here face-to-face tuition augmented the materials based learning. The students then spent some time looking at published experimental research, selecting a paper to evaluate critically. The results of this activity were also shared in a group session. Finally, the students spent half a day with a researcher who had undertaken some experimental research, discussing the design of the study, the results, and their implications for practice.

This illustrates how the teaching of a particular subject can be satisfactorily achieved using a combination of face-to-face and materials based tuition and, equally important, may be presented in a coherent framework. During the eleven days of self-directed learning, which were spaced throughout the course as dictated by the sequencing of course content, it was necessary for the teachers to make themselves available to students as and when necessary by mutual agreement. In practice, most of the contact made by students was by telephone. Students needed to feel that support was available should they require it.

Evaluation

Overall, the use of open learning materials produced a valuable bonus, in that it released a substantial amount of teacher time, some of which was used for individual tutorial sessions. Tutorials were used to support students through any problems experienced with the course content, the process of undertaking the course, or their assessed work. But more importantly, tutorials were used to help individual students to clarify their reasons for studying the course and identify their own learning goals. Because of the diversity of background of the students enrolled on the course, individual learning contracts were negotiated.

It became apparent as a result of systematic course evaluation procedures, including the use of questionnaires, that the considerable emphasis placed on self-directed learning throughout the course had enabled individual course members to feel satisfied that they had achieved their own learning objectives. In the light of this experience, it now seems inappropriate to assume that any standardised 'message' – whether it be a written or spoken one – is interpreted in exactly the same way by a group of adult students. Different students took different things away from the course, although in general terms each individual considered that she had become more professionally self-aware, had developed a more positive and, equally important, a more realistic attitude towards research. All felt better prepared to question and analyse.

Individual students who had come from diverse backgrounds with differing needs were not 'pulled' towards a set of pre-determined, and teacher-dominated objectives. Rather, they were encouraged to express their own learning needs and were guided towards the achievement of those goals. Within this framework, the responsibility must, therefore, rest largely with individual students to gauge how far their knowledge, understanding and attitudes have developed and the extent to which their goals have been met. Research is now needed to investigate whether self-directed learning based on open learning materials produces a more profound and long-lasting impact on professional practice than other modes of learning.

The philosophy of the course required a certain amount of trust. The teachers were occasionally asked whether they were worried that students might in fact be doing other things rather than studying during the study days when they were not required to be in college. Whilst one can understand the cause of this concern, experience has shown that such questions need not cause undue worry. In any case, students' concentration in the classroom also certainly lapses – students may take micro, or even macro sleeps, or they may even write their shopping lists! We must clearly move away from the unquestioned assumption that the most effective learning is classroom based, and systematically evaluate the effectiveness of different modes of teaching and learning.

One thing that did become apparent was the vastly different lengths of time individual students took to work through the open learning modules. Those able to work at a faster pace found time to follow up some of the suggestions for further reading in the time available. The majority of students commented favourably on the opportunity to retain the open learning materials for future reference and to go back over specific activities and sections of the text whenever they chose – which was sometimes after a considerable lapse of time. They also welcomed the opportunity to involve colleagues, who were not themselves following the course, in certain of the activities, and this was found to be a highly effective means of reinforcing workplace learning experiences.

It is also important that the assessment scheme of any course should correspond with the course philosophy. In line with the increased responsibility given to the students for their learning, via the use of open learning materials and individually negotiated learning contracts, students undertook a project that was open ended and individually negotiated to meet their own learning needs and which was derived from their own work area and experience.

In the final week of the course, during a visit from the ENB Education Officer who had been involved in course validation procedures, it was suggested that the students might like to consider preparing a joint statement of how they felt the course had affected their professional practice – if indeed they felt it had. The group decided that this would be a useful activity and that it would be appropriate to do it as part of the post-course day planned about four months after the end of the course. The statement they prepared is reproduced (with their permission) below:

> The course has emphasised for us the need, in the light of the UKCC Code of Professional Conduct, for an awareness of current research to be an essential factor in every individual's

competence and professional function. It is vital for each practitioner to be able to develop and use a questioning approach and self-evaluation in regard to individual competence and the recognition of limitations. To evaluate effectively, one must be aware of the knowledge available so that valid assessment of situations can be made. The ability to critique and use research findings can directly improve clinical practice and enhance the credibility of the profession.

Open learning does not exclude face-to-face teaching although often the use of learning materials replaces much of the teaching element, leaving the counselling role to be performed by the course teacher. However in this case study the open learning materials contributed to but did not replace the traditional teaching. The results of the course evaluation suggest that open learning materials can make a valuable contribution to continuing professional education programmes by complementing traditional approaches. Indeed, the economics of providing mandatory periodic refreshment courses for all registered nurses and health visitors may mean that district health authorities will have to consider using open learning materials if they are to meet the future education needs of the profession.

Looking towards the future, teachers will be able to select from a growing range of carefully prepared open learning materials. And to help teachers keep in touch with what is currently available, the ENB issues an educational resource list of open learning materials for the nursing curriculum which is regularly updated. However, new insights will only be possible if open learning materials are used in a variety of different ways and settings which are then systematically evaluated, and the results of such evaluations shared (*see,* for example, Thorpe 1988; Crotty and Bignell 1988). Only by systematically investigating whether aims have been achieved and expectations met, and by identifying both unexpected problems and opportunities afforded by the use of open learning materials, will our understanding of their effectiveness develop further.

As we have seen, a key feature of any good open learning material is its flexibility; now is the time to experiment with the flexibility offered. And as the choice of available materials continues to expand, users must learn to distinguish what is good from what is less good and choose those producers that are making the best use of the Code of Practice outlined by the MSC. Only then can we ensure that the highest possible standards of quality continue to prevail.

References

Cropley A and Kahl T 1983 Distance education and distance learning: some psychological considerations. *Distance Education* 4 (1) pp27-39

Crotty M M and Bignall A R 1988 Using a quality assurance model to evaluate ENB course 998:Teaching and assessing in clinical practice. *Nurse Education Today* 8 pp332-40

English National Board 1988 *Open and distance learning: an educational resource list of open/distance learning materials for the nursing curriculum* (This list is available from the Resource and Careers Services, 764a Chesterfield Road, Sheffield S8 0SE)

Farnish S E 1983 *Ward Sister Preparation: A Survey in Three Districts* Nursing Education Research Unit, Department of Nursing Studies, Chelsea College, London

Knowles M S 1987 Foreword. In Hodgson V E, Mann S J, and Snell R (eds.) *Beyond Distance Teaching Towards Open Learning.* The Society for Research into Higher Education and Open University Press

Lathlean J 1986 *Post Registration Courses for Qualified Nurses: An Evaluation.* Ashdale Press

Lawrence J, Maggs C, Rogers J 1988 *Interim Report on an Evaluation of the Use of Distance Learning Materials for Continuing Professional Education for Qualified Nurses, Midwives and Health Visitors.* Institute of Education, University of London

Manpower Services Commission 1988 *Ensuring Quality in Open Learning: A Handbook for Action.* Manpower Services Commission

Morgan A 1985 What shall we do about independent learning? *Teaching at a Distance* 26 pp38-45

Paley J 1986 The challenge of open learning. *Nursing Times* 82 (50) December 10 pp55-8

Perry W 1986 *Open University: A Personal Account by the First Vice-Chancellor.* Open University Press

Rogers J and Lawrence J 1987 *Continuing Professional Education for Qualified Nurses, Midwives and Health Visitors.* Ashdale Press and Austen Cornish Publishers

Stainton Rogers W 1983 Alternative uses of materials. *Teaching at a Distance* 24 pp49-54

Stainton Rogers W 1986 Changing attitudes through distance learning *Open Learning* 1 3 pp12-17

Stainton Rogers W 1987 Adapting materials for alternative use. In Thorpe M and Grugeon D (eds.) *Open Learning for Adults.* Longman

Thorpe M 1988 *Evaluating Open and Distance Learning.* Longman

United Kingdom Central Council 1987 *Discussion Paper: Mandatory Periodic Refreshment for Nurses and Health Visitors.* United Kingdom Central Council for Nursing, Midwifery and Health Visiting

13 Helping enrolled nurses

Margaret Johnston

In Oxfordshire, learning packages have been used extensively by enrolled nurses since 1986, but when the venture began, enrolled nurses had very limited understanding of what open or distance learning was all about. In this chapter I want to explain how the scheme began, who used it, where it was used, and why it was introduced in the first place. I will include a brief outline of how the scheme operated, who the facilitators were and what help was provided for the enrolled nurses planning to use the packs. The last part of the chapter will discuss the educational benefits with examples from particular packs and comments from facilitators and learners.

How the scheme began

In May 1986, at a time of increasing anxiety and uncertainty for enrolled nurses, I was appointed Nurse Teacher for Enrolled Nurses in Oxfordshire Health District to give enrolled nurses support and plan appropriate training programmes. At that time there were 685 (approximately 500 whole-time equivalent) enrolled nurses employed, although now there are considerably more. Several studies (reported in Johnston and Ross 1988) all indicated a need for more educational opportunities and there was some indication in work by Johnston and Ross (1988) of the kind of opportunities which enrolled nurses thought was appropriate. There was support from management, exemplified by the creation of my post, and articulated by the statement to the enrolled nurses by the Chief Nursing Officer: '...training will be provided to enable you to be more secure in your role and in your position in the team...' (Ross 1986, cited in Johnston and Ross 1988). However, the problem of mobilising sufficient resources remained acute. A survey by Johnston (cited in Johnston and Ross 1988) had identified a level of needs which could not possibly be met by conventional learning methods within existing resources, so the use of open learning seemed the available method which offered the greatest opportunity to the greatest number.

Enrolled nurses were beginning to show interest in up-dating and demonstrating a thirst for knowledge, yet staff shortages created difficulties when it came to releasing them regularly for courses. Some lacked confidence in returning to learning after so many years, and viewed with little enthusiasm the 'talk and chalk' approach which they expected with exams, tests, hard work and little enjoyment. The resource used to solve these problems was the independent learning pack. The range of learning packs available (with more on the way) widened access to learning opportunities and were ready to meet learners' immediate needs, for example, the *Management of Learning* pack (Continuing Nurse Education Programme 1986). Problems such as the booking of rooms, equipment, car parking and geographical separation disappeared. Making full use of what learning materials were available within an open learning structure was the only hope of beginning to meet the needs of over 600 enrolled nurses.

However, most enrolled nurses had never seen a learning package, let alone used one, so how was a scheme to be developed? A number of options were explored. First, I could encourage the enrolled nurses to buy learning packages for themselves, but generally they were unwilling to find cash for a package which might only be used once. A second option would be for wards or departments to buy packs for their enrolled nurses and others, and this sometimes happens after packs have been initially used by enrolled nurses. A third option, which I understand has been tried elsewhere, is for groups to get together to buy packs and circulate them amongst the group. The fourth option, which was the one which was eventually developed, was to buy a number of packages with money that was available from the League of Friends and trust funds, and operate a loan scheme specifically for the enrolled nurses. And although they had been reluctant to purchase, they proved eager to hire packs at a minimum cost which went towards meeting the costs of the scheme and the purchase of new packs. It was judged that this would be seen as an attractive scheme which might stimulate desire to learn, especially if support was offered, without being in any way threatening.

I decided to buy the packs which seemed most relevant to the needs of enrolled nurses and to 'hire' them out on a monthly basis, offering various degrees of support. The scheme was introduced to the users through wide discussion, handouts, and the use of demonstration packs, and it was advertised in the new quarterly newsletter *Rollcall* which was sent to all enrolled nurses employed in the NHS in Oxfordshire. In order to gather more information about open learning packs and to discuss the possibilities of using their materials, which I thought were most suitable for initial use, I visited the Distance Learning Centre (DLC) in London. The scheme has subsequently used their materials in conjunction with those of the Continuing Nurse Education Programme (CNEP) and the Open University (OU). Since this scheme was established there is much more information available about the use of learning packs, and the ENB has produced guidelines for possible use of open learning for enrolled nurses as part of the criteria towards conversion to first level nurses (English National Board 1988b).

Using packages

Teachers, facilitators (including myself) and enrolled nurses working in the District have found the published packages extremely useful. A number of enrolled nurse who were temporarily out of nursing also made use of them.They have all found the packages a useful way of 'refreshing' or providing new ideas to explore with colleagues in the workplace. There are packs to suit nurses on different parts of the register, and they accommodate nurses working in both hospital and community settings. This type of learning has proved popular with those who work unsocial hours, such as night staff, evening staff and week-end workers. 'Bank' enrolled nurses, who are expected to work in acute clinical settings using current approaches to nursing practice, have commented on the usefulness of packs to help them develop their knowledge base and skills and explore their attitudes (the use of packs for bank nurses is explored further in Chapter 14). Enrolled nurses working in comparative isolation have been able to update knowledge, widen horizons and in some instances enhance career development.

How the scheme operated

After the packs had been in use for just over two years they also became available through the District library. This eased demand for the packs held within the scheme but it is now almost impossible to monitor their use, so this account relates to the introduction of the scheme rather than the current use of packs by enrolled nurses. Once the packs were purchased they were advertised through *Rollcall* and handouts. Information was also provided on how to hire the packs and explanations about use were given when the packs were distributed. It was always emphasised that there are no age or ability boundaries as far as ENs are concerned as regards eligibility to using the packs. Packs were hired for any length of time on a monthly basis, at a cost of £2.00 per month (£0.50 for smaller packs); the first £2.00 was payable in advance and the balance at the end. The fee was waived in cases of hardship. Packs were available on a first come, first served basis. Applicants for a package which was not immediately available were put on a waiting list. There was no limit to the length of time the pack could be kept as I was anxious not to break any continuity of learning for the learner who might take longer to work through the package. The only difficulty was the problem of assessing when the pack would be available for rehire. After three months a letter was sent to enquire how the nurse was getting on with the pack. Where the packs contained activity pages for the learner to complete, our learners were asked to provide their own workbooks rather than write in the pack material. This method would avoid the costs (or the infringement of copyright) involved in copying the activity pages.

No formal or compulsory system of support was established to accompany the packs. Instead a range of options were articulated from which the student could chose, varying her choice according to her experience of open learning and the particular problems of the pack. The options for support of the learner were therefore flexible, but could be broadly categorised as:

- to hire the packs on a monthly basis with no other support and no pressure to produce work;
- to hire the pack and make use of the EN teacher or other facilitator;
- to purchase the pack and, if it was from the Distance Learning Centre, make use of their assessment facility;
- to hire the pack and produce work for the EN teacher;
- to hire the pack and work with colleagues and peers;
- to hire the pack and work with a group but without tutor input ;
- to hire the pack and work with a group with teacher input.

Whatever the option initially chosen, the EN teacher could always be called on for further assistance.

Use of facilitators/mentors

In-service sisters, clinical practice development nurses and tutors were especially helpful in providing support initially, but this role soon spread to managers, ward sisters and colleagues including other enrolled nurses. The kind of help needed varied, but in general terms the learners needed both practical help, such as explanations of how to use packs and the provision of resources such as tape recorders, and more personal help with maintaining interest and motivation. Support was provided through drop-in sessions, use of the internal mail system, regular meetings and telephone counselling – an answerphone and a radiopager made communication easier. I also found that it was important always to have a stock of handouts advertising the various packs. Regular feedback from the learners has always been encouraged but no-one has been pressurised into 'producing results'.

The pack usage

The original stock of packs included only seven titles, but within a year extra copies had been purchased of the most popular titles and a dozen or so new titles added as they became available from the producers. The subjects range right across the spectrum including those which might not be thought of as suitable for ENs such as teaching and assessing nurses and nursing research.

In the first year of operation of the system 104 packs were used, 91 were hired, and the rest were studied as part of the developmental testing programme of the producers. However, the figure for the following year was 283. These figures relate only to the scheme and do not include, for example, ENs who were working with other groups on the pack *A Systematic Approach to Nursing Care* (Open University 1984). Even within the scheme we know that many of the hired packs were shared between friends to avoid the waiting list. A number of enrolled nurses have also commented that they made use of the Nursing Times/Distance Learning Centre pullout supplements, although no figures were available.

Lessons learned

Many of the benefits of the scheme have already been highlighted but in contrast it is important to note that exclusive dependence on an open learning scheme might be counterproductive. In my experience, ENs benefit most from a variety of learning opportunities and a wide range of teaching strategies. The construction of an open learning system is only one of these strategies, but a useful and cost effective one. However, the assessment of learners is potentially more difficult and the learner might decide to skip areas of learning which seem too difficult or unmanageable. For example, one nurse who worked on a package while on night duty in a low dependency, usually quiet, area skipped the pack activities which depended on discussions with a group of colleagues as he found it logistically difficult. This obviously inhibited his learning. Where packages are used independently there is little or no contact time with a teacher and it may be difficult to measure – from the teacher's viewpoint – whether learning has taken place or to fully evaluate the success or otherwise of the packages.

Another concern is the lack of information available from the producers of packs, in particular, the absence of a grading or labelling system of packs according to difficulty. For example, *The Management of Learning* and *Interpersonal Skills* are both published by the Continuing Nurse Education Programme, but while the former is very suitable for beginners, the latter is not. Another type of coding might emphasise packs with predominantly psychomotor, affective or cognitive skills, although titles do help with this aspect to a certain extent. Some packs are also found to be more 'user-friendly' than others and although introductions varied a number of learners would have liked objectives listed more specifically. Assuming that the packs were used more or less as intended it should be comparatively easy to list at the beginning what the learner could be reasonably expected to be able to do at the end, rather than what one learner described as 'a rather flowery approach' and another called 'waffle'. A number wanted an introduction which was brief and clear but also gave indications of the demands on learners, especially where, for example, visiting a library was desirable, or particular resources such as video needed. Ideally advertising literature would indicate prereading which would help and resources which would be advantageous. In the absence of this sort of labelling the onus is very much on the scheme organiser to advise on such matters, which makes it imperative that she has a more than superficial knowledge of each pack. As more packs became available so this will make increasing demands on time.

Text was generally found to be the most suitable medium for individual use, while video-tapes, audio-tapes, tape-slide packages and computer aided material were more suited to group work as equipment was not universally available. It would appear from our experience that users of packs are unlikely to be given any time in which to do them. This contrasts with courses where time away from the working environment is usually available.

The learners

What of the learners' perspective; how did they feel about open learning? It very much depended on what pack they had chosen to do – their comments reflect the particular usefulness of that pack rather than 'open learning' as an abstract formulation. The *Management of Learning* pack (Continuing Nurse Education programme 1986), for example, evoked this eulogy:

> After being accepted for the fifty-two week conversion course, it dawned on me that it had been many years since I had had to study. I had participated in In-service Education Study Days and did an Open University distance learning pack but real studying...! it had been a while. Margaret Johnston suggested the *Management of Learning* pack. It is a continuing nurse education pack for self-improvement. What a boon it was! It taught me how to organise my learning, how to read and take in what I was reading, how to obtain useful information, improve my written work and how to use facilities available, such as the library, as a resource. It turned on a few light bulbs in the old cob-web filled brain. Joking aside, I feel the pack is a useful tool for anyone who has not participated in formal education for a

long period of time. I highly recommend it for anyone who feels their study habits may need a tune-up.

Rollcall June 1987

Obviously the fact that the pack addressed and solved the learner's immediate problem was of primary importance. Similarly, nurses who are returning from a break in service have found *Nursing Today* (Continuing Nurse Education Programme 1986) particularly useful, and nurses struggling to succeed with the local drug administration course have had the motivation to cope with *Measurement in Nursing* (Continuing Nurse Education Programme 1986).

The nurses used the packs in different ways. For example, a considerable number had chosen to involve colleagues and work together through *Interpersonal Skills* (Continuing Nurse Education Programme 1986). A typical comment was:

> *This was a pack which was better done at work with colleagues – I felt that was the best way to get maximum benefit from it. Sister is now going to purchase a pack for the ward.*

And another,

> *It helps if you have a sensitive person to assist so that you can explore ideas and discover hidden depths of your own character which may help or hinder you to be assertive without being aggressive.*

In general, comments on the packs are positive:

> *It was very good and I learned a lot about myself as well as patients.*

> *I particularly found the section on the calculation of drug dosages interesting and useful reading.*

> *Packs were very useful. I enjoyed reading them.*

> *I have enjoyed using the pack so much I would like you to send me an up to date list of all other distance learning packages you have on offer – I can't afford to buy them myself.*

It is not entirely clear whether the comments relate to the method of learning or the content – probably both – and clearly some became enamoured of the method as well as the themes:

> *I was so stimulated I am now going to take a course with the Open University called 'Health and Disease' which will contain similar points in more depth as the course you ran for us incorporating distance learning packages.*

Some idea of the sort of problems enrolled nurses have with packs can be demonstrated by looking at the experience which two groups had in testing packs for the producers. There were ENs in the group from various sites and specialties, including outside the NHS. Some found the material daunting, particularly when dealing with the theoretical component:

> *I hoped I would be able to do this and enjoy it but I'm afraid I can't set my mind to it and concentrate. I bit off more than I could chew.*

One nurse withdrew from the group. She worked in an isolated setting and seemed to get little support from managers. While she obviously needed open learning opportunities she couldn't yet cope with the isolation of learning as well as the isolation of her work.

An important issue shown up by the testing was the ENs preference for 'concrete' material, with a tendency towards 'right or wrong' answers. Packs like *Measurement in Nursing* were generally liked, whereas less specific topics were better dealt with in groups of peers and colleagues and possibly teacher led. Some learners remained unhappy without a teacher:

> *You miss the rewards such as praise of a tutor which you might receive when you master something you have found to be especially difficult and although friends may say 'that's nice' it never seems to mean quite the same.*

The timing of some of the testing caused difficulties, being just before Christmas. Not only were there staff shortages on wards with sickness compounding the taking of annual leave and the preparations for Christmas on the wards, but in their own time the learners were involved in Christmas shopping and 'pre-Christmas tension'. And personal timing can always go wrong – one tester's husband was unexpectedly hospitalised and subsequently needed care on discharge.

Possibilities for the future

There are a number of developments in open learning which offer interesting developments in the future – the use of computer aided learning, for example, or the growth in independent study incorporating open learning as a respectable route to academic qualifications (Dixon 1987). However, as far as enrolled nurses are concerned, one of the most exciting developments has been the proposed use of learning packages within the second to first level nurse conversion courses and courses for the conversion of the second level specialist qualification to the first level one. The UKCC in its paper: *The enrolled nurse and preparation for entry to a first level part of the UKCC's register* (1988) stated:

> The UKCC is extremely concerned and aware of the difficulties experienced by large numbers of enrolled nurses in securing a place on existing conversion or bridging courses.

The circular set out new approaches to creating greater flexibility and increasing opportunities. The programme, which may be undertaken on a full or part time basis may be a specially designed course or comprise an individually designed range of approved learning activities. These activities could include face-to-face teaching on a day release basis, learning at a distance using learning packs, contract learning and planned modules from existing courses. However, for the proposals to be realised in full, many more tailor made learning packs would be required. Nevertheless, the identified need should provide a challenge for those involved in the development of learning packs.

Evaluation

This chapter has provided an overview of my experiences when introducing an open learning scheme to enrolled nurses over a two year period. My thoughts at the end of that period were that open learning opportunities are here to stay and that it need not be only *nursing* learning packs which are used within nursing education. This type of learning lends itself to credit accumulation systems which will be increasingly prevalent in the future. I do not feel, however that this type of learning should replace other teaching strategies and there is a need for a variety of options.

I found that it could be a useful non-threatening method to offer to groups of mixed ability and confidence, and older age groups in particular, but only if introduced in a proper manner bearing in mind how some found the packs daunting at first glance. I propose that more information about the packs be made available by the producers, including some kind of grading system and offering more information about the level of knowledge expected of the user. Useful articles to read which are required or found to be useful when doing the pack should be included.

All libraries should be encouraged to keep a wide selection of packs. I measured popularity by the numbers used and the length of time packs were kept. As there was a hire fee, I assumed that it was unlikely that enrolled nurses would ask for packs or keep them indefinitely if they weren't being used. However I didn't make any checks on use as I thought these would be intrusive.

Finally, educational benefits far outweigh drawbacks in my opinion. An enrolled nurse asked me recently what I would be when I finished learning. My reply: *'Dead!'*. We need to change the attitudes which suggest that learning to be a good nurse is a fixed term contract, but if education *is* to be a life long experience, teaching strategies need to be attractive, user-friendly and accessible. In my experience, open learning schemes can meet this specification. They create the potential for facilitating Project 2000, the recommendations of which include the suggestion that '...opportunities for continuing education be explored and developed to help retain the confidence of present enrolled nurses and to enhance their expertise.' (United Kingdom Central Council 1987).

References

Continuing Nurse Education 1986 *Management of Learning*

Continuing Nurse Education 1986 *Nursing Today*

Continuing Nurse Education 1986 *Measurement in Nursing*

Continuing Nurse Education 1986 *Interpersonal Skills*

Dixon K 1987 *Implementing Open Learning in Local Authority Institutions*. Further Education Unit and Open Learning Branch of Manpower Services Commission, 2nd Edition

English National Board 1987 *Criteria to be examined when considering courses with an open learning component for approval by the ENB*. English National Board for Nursing, Midwifery and Health Visiting OLWG/14/87

English National Board 1988a *Working group on opportunities for enrolled nurses (general)*. English National Board for Nursing, Midwifery and Health Visiting RMHLV/FF 31.5.1988

English National Board 1988b *Spectrum of opportunities for enrolled nurses*. Paper 5. Guidelines for recognition of previous learning within flexible schemes for second to first level nurse conversion. Circular 1988/67/RMHLV English National Board for Nursing, Midwifery and Health Visiting

Johnston M, Ross M 1988 *The Way Forward. Clinical development for enrolled nurses – a guide for managers.* Oxfordshire Health Authority

Johnston M, Moss A (eds.) 1986 *Rollcall* A newsletter for enrolled nurses in Oxfordshire. Oxfordshire Health Authority, September

Johnston M, Moss A (eds.) 1987 *Rollcall* A newsletter for enrolled nurses in Oxfordshire. Oxfordshire Health Authority, June

Johnston M, Fitzgerald M, Hoffman I 1988 Drug giving for enrolled nurses *Nursing Times* Vol 84 No 2 Jan pp13-9

Johnston M 1988 Developing Potential *Nursing Times* Vol 84 No 48 Nov pp34-7

Open University 1984 *A Systematic Approach to Nursing Care.* Open University Press

United Kingdom Central Council 1987 *Project 2000: The final proposals.* Project Paper 9. United Kingdom Central Council for Nursing, Midwifery and Health Visiting

United Kingdom Central Council 1988 *The enrolled nurse and preparation for entry to a first level part of the UKCC register.* United Kingdom Central Council for Nursing, Midwifery and Health Visiting PS&D/88/05

14 Helping bank nurses

Wendy Green

Nurses who do not hold standard contracts with a health authority but who work intermittently through a nurse bank are particularly hard to reach through conventional teaching programmes. People who, for whatever reason, cannot cope with regular working hours are unlikely to be able to cope with the timing of most conventional courses. However, the use of learning materials in conjunction with some regular meetings has proved very successful in meeting their educational needs. This brief account describes the use of open learning with bank nurses in one health authority. However, in order to understand why open learning is particularly suitable for this group it is necessary to understand how a nurse bank works and how bank nursing has changed in recent years.

The nurse bank

When the nurse bank was started there were two main aims. First, to give an opportunity to married women with family commitments to get back into hospital, working infrequent hours on a casual basis, and second, to help staff the hospitals, filling empty lines and improving the standard of nursing care for the patients. At the beginning of the scheme the nurses recruited were supernumerary until they had familiarised themselves with the hospital and new techniques and procedures and they were all given a basic idea of procedures in the School of Nursing before starting work. In addition, they were required to attend a course or lectures which included drug administration, intravenous infusion, cardiac arrest procedures, preparation for tests and X-rays and CSSD.

In the mid-1970s, this preparation for returning to practice and to work as a bank nurse was adequate as change in the organisation and delivery of care was slow. New nursing knowledge had yet to explode on the clinical scene and nursing research was in its infancy. But slowly, towards the end of the 1970s, outside influences and local circumstances began to change the situation. In particular, as their numbers increased and the nurses themselves became more experienced, bank staff began to be used in crisis situations. However, it was still assumed that, from the experience of working in a variety of different fields of nursing, the nurses would increase their knowledge and skills and be able to work in more specialised fields such as the renal transplant unit or theatres. Many bank nurses attended lectures in the hospitals where they worked and some were included in weekly or bi-weekly ward meetings.

At the end of 1975 the whole NHS was hit by a financial crisis. The effect this had on the nurse bank was that the nurses could only be used when specifically requested by a line manager to cover staff shortages. This meant that the majority of nurses were requested for night-duty or to work on the private ward or specialist units. Many bank nurses resigned to find other work, which made it increasingly difficult to fill the requests for cover. A recruitment drive became necessary and it was also proposed to run a course of lectures requested by bank nurses. In 1979 concern was expressed by bank nurses that they were given little in-service training and because of ward work-load it was difficult for the permanent staff to give them help. Some bank nurses left because of unacceptably high levels of anxiety. The outcome was the appointment of one full-time and one part-time clinical teacher specifically for bank nurses. They were to be responsible for:

- the orientation of new bank nurses, including working alongside them
- offering support in the clinical areas
- arranging monthly lectures which bank nurses would attend in their own time
- arranging one or two-day courses in specialised fields such as ITU and renal work.

Although the bank nurses much appreciated the orientation and support in the clinical areas and being up-dated in current nurse thinking, the monthly lectures were not well attended. The main reasons given for this were inconvenient timing of the lectures and the high cost of travel to the lectures. The cost of travel was met by a trust fund and the timing was adjusted but as the pace of change within nursing accelerated problems remained. Bank nursing, although still organised centrally, is now paid for mainly by the individual hospitals or units who hold their own nursing budget. This means that bank nurses can only be paid for out of funded posts, thus there must be a vacancy before a bank nurse can be used by the hospital. The expectation of the nurse manager is therefore for a qualified nurse, accountable for her own practice. The nurse will most likely be used in a busy, fraught situation with little or no help or support as this account shows:

> *My first night on duty the enrolled nurse was very understanding. My second night on duty I was on a male surgical ward and 'in charge'. There were ten post-ops that day, seven patients had metri-sets and two had CVP lines which I had never seen before. There were also IV drugs to give and I was on duty with a second year student, her first night on the ward. It was a terrible night which I will never forget. I had been out of nursing for fourteen years and said so. There were similar nights when I was in charge, fifteen out of forty six nights in fact. Often out of these fifteen nights a third year student nurse wrote the Kardex, but I was actually responsible because I was trained. After five nights I joined the RCN.*
>
> A bank nurse

The bank nurse is also seen by a hard pressed manager as a mobile resource and the nurse could well be moved once, if not twice, in a shift. She seldom has a choice of where she works and cannot expect continuity of experience:

> *I would be willing to commit myself to duties a month ahead if it meant I could stay on one ward for that time.*
>
> *While I understand how the situation may arise, I do very much resent turning up for duty to find I am asked to go somewhere else.*
>
> *I work night duty and never know which ward I will be working on until I arrive, even when I am booked to work on a certain level I can be moved to another.*
>
> Three bank nurses

The bank nurse

The bank nurse herself has changed since the mid-1970s as a result of both social and professional pressures. A profile of the 'typical' bank nurse would show these characteristics:

- female, as very few men work for the bank
- between thirty and forty years old and having been out of

nursing for three to ten years
- has two children between three and ten years old
- is possibly a one-parent family
- needs to work for financial reasons and is less likely to work just to 'keep in touch'
- recognises the need to belong to a professional organisation
- recognises the importance of continuing education.

Although in the past, a majority of bank nurses worked to keep in touch, with a view to returning to part-time or full-time work when their domestic commitments allowed, today they are much more likely to work for financial reasons to supplement the family income and pay for necessities such as the mortgage. Night and weekend work, which is better paid, is always booked up first. These nurses, therefore, *have* to work and foresee that they will want to continue to work in the future, so they know they must cope with the challenges presented by present day practice. They recognise their vulnerability and employ a variety of strategies to cope with it including education.

> *I have been away from full-time nursing for three and a half years, but returned to working for the bank between babies. I think it would be nice to have some reorientation in all fields, as most of all it gives confidence again, since things change so quickly – drugs, etc.*

> A bank nurse

> *I work as a midwife for the nurse bank and would very much like to be informed of any courses or lectures that the permanent staff attend. I would appreciate any help to keep me up-to-date in midwifery.*

> A bank midwife

Learning needs

It is evident that as both nursing and the bank nurse have changed and developed considerably over the past decade the learning needs of the bank nurse have also changed. Whereas in the mid-1970s when the nurse bank was first set up the bank nurse was supernumerary until she had regained her old skills, by the mid-1980s bank nurses were never supernumerary and were often found in a crisis situation with few other trained staff around with the time or patience to retrain the unsure bank nurse. She must therefore be competent and confident before she sets foot on a ward, particularly in specialised units:

> *Going to specialised units makes life more difficult when you've never had specialised training. Often one feels like a*

> *spare part not knowing the unit and spending twice as long doing something, even looking for items.*

> A bank nurse

Another problem bank nurses face is the varied use to which they are put when on duty. This may range from being an auxiliary or 'pair of hands' through to being the only qualified nurse on duty and therefore being in charge of running the ward and being wholly accountable.

> *There is an attitude that the bank nurse is just a pair of hands, especially amongst student nurses who do not give the bank nurse credit for being a qualified nurse and treat them as auxiliaries until a crisis arrives when they expect you to sort it out for them.*

> A bank nurse

However the largest and most common learning need identified by bank nurses is the ever changing technology and the need to be conversant with a whole range of often quite sophisticated equipment:

> *At one point in the evening I was asked by a doctor to set up a cardiac monitor on a patient. In my book this was a non-nursing duty. Certainly neither in my training nor at any time since have I been instructed as to how to set one up. I explained this to the doctor who replied 'ring up the night sister and get her to do it then'.*

> A bank nurse

The change to individualised care and the use of the nursing process also confuses many who were trained in the task allocation system. Ten years ago she could have matched the tasks she was assigned with her level of confidence, but today she will be asked to look after a group of patients, reading and understanding their care plans and carrying out the care prescribed largely unsupervised. Although many bank nurses find this interesting and rewarding, others find the inability to offer continuity of care and the difficulty of giving advice and help to friends and relatives when you don't even know the ward is frustrating.

Though of less immediate concern, many bank nurses who have been out of touch for a few years find the changes in management structures disconcerting. Recognising individuals who might appear on the ward can be worrying for a bank nurse, but more importantly she needs to understand the procedures for dealing with problems or complaints.

But the most overwhelming concern felt by bank nurses is their lack of knowledge of nursing itself, especially as they see the body of knowledge continually growing and becoming less accessible to them. They find that they can no longer rely on past knowledge and experience but need to continually question their practice and strive to make their decisions soundly based. This leads them to increase their demands for education in general, although each of them has particular worries and concerns ranging from 'the principles of neurosurgical nursing' to 'an intensive course including work on the wards and lectures on drugs, equipment, machinery and the latest treatment of pressure sores.'

Planning a programme

While there is no doubt that the bank nurses have considerable learning needs, they also have considerable problems in meeting them. These problems lie with both the resources available and the bank nurse herself. In Oxfordshire we are more fortunate than many other health authorities in that we have one and a half bank nurse teachers, although this must be set against the bank nurse total of 300 (although the total number 'on the bank' is about 600, about half are nurses with permanent contracts who are working overtime, often in their own work areas).

The bank nurses themselves represent a challenge, partly because many of them have had extensive periods out of nursing and most are only available for short periods during school hours each week and sometimes only during term time. But most importantly, they work right across the spectrum of specialities each of which has a complex and ever changing knowledge base. However, on the 'plus' side, many of the bank nurses are highly motivated and bring a wealth of 'life experience' into the learning situation.

In Oxfordshire, we usually plan the learning programme on a termly basis although we try to provide a balanced experience over the whole year. The bank nurses are encouraged to ask for topics and ideas also come from permanent staff in the clinical areas, a recent example being the need to train bank nurses to use new equipment for measuring blood glucose.

From years of working with bank nurses a philosophy has evolved regarding their basic needs which states that every bank nurse:

- is a unique individual with unique learning needs
- is a stable mature person with life experiences to enhance the learning situation
- has a right to up-to-date knowledge and skills

- can have her learning needs met in a variety of ways
- is adaptable and flexible and can respond to changing situations
- lacks confidence and in some cases may lack competence
- needs peer support.

With these beliefs in mind four broad aims were agreed for the educational programme:

- to equip the nurse with relevant knowledge and skills to enable her to cope with the demands of a variety of work situations
- to create a forum for nurses to meet to exchange ideas and share problems and pleasures of work
- to introduce the nurse to a range of learning methods
- to encourage the nurse to work as independently as possible in meeting her own learning needs.

An ideal programme would allow each nurse to learn at her own pace, in her own time, in her own place, with material that is relevant to her particular situation. Such a programme would accommodate many of the problems of travel, child minding, different levels of knowledge, different rates of learning and the motivation to learn. There are many resources the bank nurse can draw upon to meet her learning needs, for example, in-house lectures, study days and courses, and diploma and degree courses at the local polytechnics and university, but the most important resources are open learning packs. It is the open learning scheme which will most meet the needs and problems of the bank nurse because:

- she can select a topic which interests her and is relevant to her current work
- she can work at her own pace and not feel embarrassed or threatened by others with more knowledge then herself
- she can work where it suits her, this may be in her own home so that she does not have to spend time and money travelling, but she can also fit the studying around the demands of children and domestic duties.

In order to give the bank nurses access to open learning materials, copies of all the packs produced have been placed in the hospital library and are available for loan for a month at a time. However, many nurses want a more structured system including group sessions, so the packs are used within a framework of group meetings. To date, group work has been mainly based on *A Systematic Approach to Nursing Care* (Open University 1984), *Mental Health Problems in*

Old Age (Open University 1988) and *Sources of Knowledge* (DLC 1987).

What, according to the bank nurses are the advantages? The 'classic' open learning advantages of studying at a pace, place and time convenient to the learner are clearly important:

> *...They allow me to do constructive study in my own time and particularly provide a lot of information that I don't have the time to go looking for.*

> *One can recap at leisure.*

> *Because I can work systematically through the pack at my own speed, recapping when necessary, when I can.*

> *I can study in my own time, refer to the audiotape whenever necessary...*

> Bank nurses

But while they are generally very impressed by the materials used they do have some problems with them, concerning both the level of the material and the topics they cover:

> *...Also find that a gap in updating technical knowledge and specific nursing care of disease...usually these are the things which cause greatest anxiety as a bank nurse.*

> *Some of the articles I find too academic/statistical...I had thought there would be more case histories and pointers on how to help/deal with patients with mental problems on a more practical level.*

> *Because its done away from work area or colleagues not always able to apply it to the work area.*

> *The packs include theory and suggestions and methods on applying this in clinical practice.*

> Bank nurses

Clearly the bank nurses want to use their educational opportunities to increase their practice competencies but find that some learning materials are inadequate. This is in part an accurate reflection of the existing learning packs but probably also reflects a lack of conviction that coping with stress, learning assertiveness, etc. are nursing competencies.

However, many of the bank nurses are very keen to participate in group work related to the learning materials:

> *It is preferable to learn in a group atmosphere; it stimulates one's interest more throwing ideas around with others...*

> *It is interesting having other people's views of the same topic.*
>   Bank nurses

However, they prefer to deal directly with the content of the packs by, for example, going over interesting activities or comparing their notes with others, rather than to move into new areas of content not dealt with in the pack. It must be remembered that learning has to fit into lives full of other subjects and bank nurses appreciate a very straightforward structure within which to work:

> *..in some the group work is not related to the actual subject you have been working on, this is frustrating.*

> *In workbook mention should be made of pages in another book for reference – too vague.*
>   Bank nurses

And because the timing of group activities is sometimes related more to full-time nurse learners than to part-timers, they often find the timing of the course too fast, although from the perspective of the tutor it is important to keep some momentum up or attendance dies away:

> *I do not find I have enough time to do them thoroughly.*

> *Not enough study time from work or in between sessions for time to take in or to do the work.*

> *Sometimes they are too long and detailed for the time most bank nurses have in between sessions to read and answer questions.*

> *They give the addled brain extra time to interpret new ideas, take on board new terminology, and longer to digest it than one would have in a straight lecture. Group work with other people's experience contributions is stimulating and encouraging BUT the study time for addled brains, busy mums, part time bank nurses is over optimistic.*
>   Bank nurses

So bank nurses find working through these packs both a challenge and a stimulation. However, it is often difficult for them to relate the knowledge to particular clinical situations because they have no consistency in where they work. Sometimes staff in clinical areas are not always helpful or supportive when bank nurses question practice in relation to the theories they have found in the learning materials. Their biggest frustration is being unable to change what they see or to introduce new ideas into the work situation to improve patient care.

Conclusion

The normal provision of continuing professional education within a health authority is mostly geared to the needs of the permanent full-time staff who are allowed to attend sessions in working time and who have a claim on training budgets. However, open learning packs used creatively and with imagination by continuing education staff could go a long way to ensure that the learning needs of this large and somewhat neglected group of nurses are met in a more structured way. Many of the bank nurses came into work through a return to practice programme and open learning can be equally useful with these nurses who have very similar problems to bank nurses.

Such schemes will clearly be a sound investment for the health authority as the bank nurse lays down foundations for future professional development that will enable her to assume more responsibility for patient care in the future. Although bank nurses can give limited time to nursing at this stage in their lives, they are very likely to move into full time posts when their circumstances change.

References

Clark E 1987 *Sources of Nursing Knowledge.* Distance Learning Centre, South Bank Polytechnic

Murray S 1978 Back to Nursing *Nursing Times.* June 1 pp904-5

Open University 1984 *A Systematic Approach to Nursing Care.* Open University Press

Open University 1988 *Mental Health Problems in Old Age.* Open University Press

Williams S 1985 Investing in the Bank *Senior Nurse* Vol 2 No 6 Feb 13 pp8-9

The quotations from bank nurses are taken from the nurse bank files, from two unpublished surveys of bank nurses undertaken in October 1979 and June 1986, and from course evaluation documents completed in 1989. All data is from Oxfordshire Health Authority.

15 Highland Health Board: a coordinated scheme

Chris Wakeling

Open learning systems can be developed from any college setting providing education and training for the nursing profession. The two prerequisites for successful transition are, first, especially developed in-house expertise, and second, carefully scheduled forward planning. In this chapter, I shall describe why and how such a scheme was introduced from 1985 onwards by the Highland College of Nursing and Midwifery for a number of specifically designated staff in both pre-registration and post-registration areas.

The Highland College of Nursing and Midwifery: pre 1985

The College, situated in Inverness, serves the Highland Health Board area and that of the Western Isles. The geography is vast, larger than that of Wales, but the population is small, about 250,000. There are 21 hospitals with a total bed complement of 2,072 and a hospital registered nursing population of 1,400. There are also 19 Health Centre Clinics with 233 community registered primary health care staff. Prior to 1985, the College already had a history of undertaking experimental basic training for its establishment of 370 students but within a conventional approach to education. The comprehensive modular training programme had a two and a half-year generic component and a half-year specialist (general, mental health, mental handicap) nursing component. Students chose their specialist component just after the end of the second year of training and therefore had experience of theory and practice and were aware of their own abilities and preferences. (Many chose two specialist components and were, therefore, able to register on two parts of the Register for the General Nursing Council for Scotland, after three and a half years training.) This experiment allowed teaching and service staff to develop clinically oriented modules in which theory supported the practice and utilised current research. The establishment was thirty nurse teachers (Clinical Teachers and Tutors) who taught in the College and practiced side-by-side with students in designated ward settings; they are grouped in specialist teaching teams. In 1982, the General Nursing Council for Scotland developed a semi-comprehensive training on a modular basis, with the generic stage being eighteen months, and the specialist being eighteen months. Therefore, we were able to carry forward the expertise gained in our experimental course to the revised national system. The culmination of this within the College was a recognition of the need for specialist teachers who were experts in a particular area of practice and who could, therefore, work closely with clinical colleagues offering these colleagues a 'consultancy' resource for the day-to-day work and in-service training in conjunction with Clinical Nurse Managers.

The in-service training that was developed consisted of half-day and day sessions, frequently in outlying hospitals, with teaching staff participating as peripatetic teachers. Although there were national curricula for post-basic courses under the auspices of the Committee for Clinical Nursing Studies, no courses had been developed in the Highlands. Seconding staff outwith the Highlands on such courses was a major drain because of the expenses and consequently few places were being made available; however the result was a loss of staff to promotion outside the area.

1985: Why open and distance learning?

By 1985, interest in open and distance learning systems was coming to the fore in vocational educational systems generally, stimulated by, for example, the Manpower Services Commission Open Tech initiative. More locally, in 1984, the College staff had participated in the development of a major shared training initiative for nursing and social work staff in relation to service to people with learning difficulties. The preparation of this project opened a series of dialogues with colleges and individuals with existing expertise in the field of open learning. Two major documents, *Continuing Education for the Nursing Profession in Scotland* (Scottish Home and Health Department 1981) and *Guidelines for Continuing Education Professional Studies 1 and 2* (National Board for Scotland, February 1985), were indicating the need for a structured post-basic education system available to all nursing staff throughout Scotland.

These triggers, together with the low availability of post-basic courses in the North of Scotland, led quickly to a recognition that the creation of an acceptable educational system for qualified staff could only be undertaken on an open learning basis using materials at a distance from the College. At that stage, there was no particular plan to make changes in the pre-registration programme. Recognising, however, the need to prepare future trained staff to utilise open learning systems, it became clear to us that we would also have to introduce open learning at pre-registration level.

Key principles adopted

Early in 1985, therefore, the decision was taken by myself and senior colleagues within the College to explore the feasibility of developing post-registration training for staff in the Highlands and Western Isles. We were committed to and have been guided by several key principles:

- Our own College staff required preparation in terms of training and commitment
- The programme had to be consistent in strategy terms with the objectives of the respective Health Boards
- Service staff at senior level had to be in agreement in principle and prepared to commit financial and management resources
- The overall aim of the post-registration programme had to be designed to demonstrably improve practice and its outcomes in terms of patient care
- It was not intended that this would be a cheap approach to providing education and training in terms of either finance, time or manpower and this was to be made explicit to all concerned.

The strategy

The strategy was scheduled to begin in 1987 and was designed to offer programmes to 170 Registered Nurses each year. The Registered Nurses would be up to and including the grade of Clinical Nurse Manager and from hospital situations. Community Nurses and Midwives were excluded at this stage because they all had post-registration qualifications. This number of students represents 12.5 per cent of the workforce. The best available materials were to be used for the scheme and three approaches to providing materials relevant to local learning needs were used. First, learning materials were bought and used without adaptation from the Open University (*The Systematic Approach to Nursing Care*). Next, we purchased and adapted materials from the Distance Learning Centre at South Bank Polytechnic and the Continuing Nurse Education Programme at Barnet College. Lastly, we are now in the process of authoring and designing our own materials for the Professional Studies Diploma of the National Board for Scotland.

Four courses are to be offered in total: the Continuing Education course for Second Level Nurses; Consolidation for First Level Nurses;

the Diploma in Nursing, a Distance Learning Centre course for which the Highland College of Nursing and Midwifery acts as the Local Study Centre (*see* Chapter 11 for a discussion of local study centres) for Clinical Nurse Managers, Charge Nurses and Staff Nurses; and Professional Studies I and II for First Level Registered Nurses. Figure 15.1 shows the time scale for the implementation, which is currently running to schedule.

We are starting courses with fixed entry dates and hope to move to individual flexible entry on at least some of the courses. All students are able to define their own study venue and study pattern. They are tending to use home as their base for reading and written work but to use the work setting for practical work. All five senior managers agreed at Unit level to release staff undertaking any course on a basis of 20 per cent of the required study time irrespective of the total number of hours on any course. This, therefore, can vary from ten hours to six weeks in any year, depending on the type of course.

Facilitators and tutors

It was recognised that each of the learners would require, in addition to a College facilitator, a 'mentor' at the place of work, who would normally be their line manager, but who would themselves require training to support the students in open learning. An open learning pack on teaching, learning supervision and assessment is, therefore, included (*see* Figure 15.1) within Professional Studies I and II and is also available, free standing, on an open learning basis to all mentors.

Tutor functions for the four courses and 170 students are standardised. The tutors provide individual telephone tuition for students at a distance and face-to-face tutorials both in College and at the student's place of work. They also provide group opportunities for learners in terms of induction and, during courses, for experiential learning. These may be in College or hospital-based as appropriate to the objectives. All cognitive work is provided by learning materials. Applying theory towards greater practice competence is evaluated by the mentor and the tutor together in individual work settings. The tutor also assesses the theoretical component of the work towards pass/fail. Eventually, the staff team who will provide the tutorial support will comprise nine tutors on or above the grade of Senior Tutor. These tutors will each have particular expertise, for example, Health Education, Research in Nursing, Care of the Elderly, etc. This additional workload will be catered for by adjusting current working practice. Within the staff, there is a commitment to assist in the development and progress of clinical colleagues who will then be more able to teach, supervise and assess the students of basic training. Additionally, the system is under the direct day-to-day management of the Deputy Director of Nurse

H

Course	1987	1988	1989	1990	1991
A Continuing education for second level registered nurses	Commencement --September 10 weeks for 3 Open Learning packs 4 Groups per annum		——— 40 students per annum ——— →		
B Consolidation 2 week in-College course for first level registered nurses commenced in 1986 4 Courses per annum	80 students per annum conventional ↓		(converted to Open Learning in 1989)	20 students per annum converted	
C Diploma in Nursing	Commencement --September Highland College of Nursing & Midwifery local study centre for University of London		——— 10 students each year of a three year course ——— →		
D Professional Studies I and II		September ——— Commence preparation Professional Studies I		January – Commence Course Professional Studies I March – Commence preparation for Professional Studies II	September ---Commence Professional Studies II
E Tutor/counsellor and Facilitator/supervisor/ mentor Open Learning Pack		June--- Commence preparation	June Commence course	To be undertaken as required by registered nurses acting as facilitators, etc.	

Figure 15.1 Timescale for continuing education

Education, and the Director of Nurse Education chairs the Continuing Education Sub-Committee of the Statutory Local Highland and Western Isles Training Committee. The administrative and clerical support is equivalent to approximately one whole-time equivalent, but is allocated within the total resource of the College.

Development of the strategy: 1985-1987

We recognised early in 1985 that we were embarking on a process of change affecting the College, employed nursing staff, the managers and members of two Health Boards and the national validating body. Change, therefore, had to be planned and systematic. Five phases, overlapping in time, occurred.

The first of these was our own learning phase as College Director and staff members. I learned about open learning systems personally over a period of several years prior to 1985, and see my own responsibility as being able to identify and analyse its potential to meet local training needs up to and beyond the year 2000. I was then able to release my Deputy Director, himself an Open University graduate, as indeed am I, to reexamine the methods and technologies of open learning systems by visiting centres of excellence, attending courses and conferences, and seeking personal consultation with national experts.

We were given substantial assistance by particular experts from the Open University, the Distance Learning Centre, and Social Work Education Department, and these individuals subsequently assisted us with our second phase, that of selling the concept of local continuing education on this approach. At this time, we were selling the ideas to target groups – our own College staff, service managers, our Local Training Committee, and, both for funding and validation purposes, the National Board for Scotland. Much of the selling was undertaken by face-to-face discussions and informally at College Staff Study Days, visiting local hospitals and talking with officers of the National Board. Additionally, two key events were mounted – a one day seminar for college staff and nurse managers on the basic principles of open learning, and a follow-up seminar on applicability and feasibility.

The third phase of negotiation overlapped the others; it took place with college staff and with the managers at the seminar and formally with the Local Training Committee for the establishment of a Continuing Education Sub-Committee. We wrote finally to the National Board for Scotland seeking funding for the developmental and operational phases. We were also at that stage to have formal discussions with the bodies who subsequently sold materials and offered their courses under our auspices.

Course	Student group	Student numbers		Open learning pack costs		Replacement costs related to study days	Travelling and subsistence to be paid by units student distribution		Cost totals per annum £	Hidden college costs/tutorial staff etc
		Per group	Groups per annum	Per student	Per annum		Per	Group/Annum		
A	Second Level Registered Nurses	10	4	3 Open learning packs at £20 per pack = £60	for 40 students = £2,400	5 x 3 hours study sessions per student at £4.50 per hour = £2,700	Raigmore Mental Health Southern Northern	3 – 12 2 – 12 2 – 8 2 – 8	2,400 2,700	£2,494
B	First Level Registered Nurses	20	4	Nil	Nil	NB Taken from costs submitted by Directors of Nursing Services ⟵—— £40,800 ——⟶	Raigmore Mental Health Southern Northern	6 – 24 6 – 24 4 – 16 4 – 16	40,800	£4,147
C	First Level Registered Nurses	10	3	Course cost = £350 + university fee = £80 Total – £430 (3 year costs for 1 student = £1,290)	Cost for 30 students = £12,900	30 students for 4 sessions each per annum = 720 hours. Each session 6 hours at £5.50 per hour = £3,960	Raigmore Mental Health Southern Northern	3 – 9 3 – 9 2 – 6 2 – 6	12,900 3,960	Tutorial costs met by polytechnic income = £1,002
	Total numbers 150			Cost per person £418			Total costs		£62,760	

Figure 15.2 Budget for continuing education for registered nurses

The fourth phase was that of agreement and commitment. In December 1986, the Higland and Western Isles Local Training Committee established the Continuing Education Steering Committee. In April 1987, the National Board for Scotland agreed to funding a post of Senior Tutor – Open Learning at Senior Nurse 4 Grade. The five Directors of Nursing Services gave their commitment for the release of staff to undertake continuing education. I committed part of my annual budget to the development and running of the courses. From 1988/89, the Highland Health Board committed a sum of £30,000 to service toward replacement hours for seconded staff and from 1989/90, a sum of £30,000 to the College. Future financial development for the College has been agreed in principle by the Chief Area Nursing Officers of the Highland and Western Isles Health Boards.

The fifth phase has been that of development and this commenced with the appointment of the tutor post funded by the National Board for Scotland. The development team is managed by the Deputy Director of Nurse Eucation and overviewed by myself and comprises the Deputy, the Senior Tutor (Open Learning), Senior Tutor Health Education Facilitator, Senior Tutor Research Adviser and administrative support. Development comprises the writing of course programmes; the creation of the administrative systems; preparation of College staff; developmental testing of learning materials; and creation of evaluation processes. This is an on-going process which will continue into the future.

Finance

I set out with the premise that to create the programme of continuing education would be expensive. Outlined in Figure 15.2 is the cost analysis chart developed for the first four years for the Highland scheme; indicating in 1988/9 that there is a shortfall in financial provision of £2,760, taking account of the two commitments by the Health Board of £30,000 each to Service and college respectively. Had the College costs been included the shortfall would have increased by £6,641 to £9,401. (These costs do not take into account the overheads for the college.)

However, the allocation to date is adequate to maintain our committed phasing schedule. The figures assume that tutoring costs and much of the developmental costs can be absorbed within the existing annual college budget. It has to be recognised that this sum represents the cost of creating and delivering three new courses for the area from new. No paradigm exists for costing conventional courses of continuing education nursing in Scotland let alone open learning systems. Certainly, tutoring costs would not be absorbed in the same

College Costs for One 10 Day Course
Course B

TUTORIAL HOURS*

15 hours of SN3 time @ £11.08 + £5.54 = (£3.32 on cost) £19.94	£	249
15 hours of SN4 time @ £10.25 + £5.12 = (£3.74 on cost) £18.44	£	230
30 hours of Grade I time @ £ 9.09 + £4.54 = (£2.72 on cost) £16.36	£	409
On costs @ 20%	£	177
	£1,065	

ADMINISTRATION COSTS

Secretarial time – letters – programmes – photocopying	£	120
Course Total	£1,185	

COURSES RUN IN THE FINANCIAL YEAR:

May 1988	10 day course	£1,185
August 1988	10 day course	£1,185
December 1988	5 day course	£ 592
February 1989	10 day course	£1,185
Total College cost for CONSOLIDATION COURSES		£4,147

* Tutorial hours are charged at 1.5 times the hourly rate + 20% on costs.
This covers preparation time and teaching time.

Figure 15.3 Consolidation courses for registered nurses

way as has occurred in the development described. As seen in Figure 15.2, Course B taught in college is expensive because of replacement costs. Travel and subsistence, the absorbed college costs, shown itemised in Figure 15.3, cost £4,147 at 1988/89 prices, making the total cost £44,947 (exclusive of college overheads!).

We are currently adapting the consolidation course to an open learning format. Figures 15.4 and 15.5 show the predicted costs for 80 students a year.

Comparing the costs for course B on Figures 15.2, 15.4 and 15.5, it can be seen that there are noticeable savings.

Course	Student group	Student numbers		Open learning pack costs		Replacement costs related to study days	Travelling and subsistence to be paid by units student distribution	Cost totals per annum £	Hidden college costs/ tutorial staff etc
		Per group	Groups per annum	Per student	Per annum		Per Group/Annum		
3 by Open Learn-ing	First Level Registered Nurses	25	3	3 Open learning packs at £25 per pack = £75	for 80 students = £6,000	4 x 3 hour study sessions per student at £5.50 per hour = £65 for 80 students = £5,280	Raigmore 6 – 24 Mental Health 6 – 24 Southern 4 – 24 Northern 4 – 24 Travel & Subsistence would be minimal as tutors would be peripatetic where necessary.	6,000 5,280	2,959
							Total Costs	£11,280	

Figure 15.4 Predicted budget for continuing education for registered nurses

Recently, we have developed an open learning study pack of thirty hours study time. The literature search, authoring and testing were undertaken by a Senior Tutor in three months. The cost is therefore 25 per cent of salary with 20 per cent on-cost plus thirty hours of typing using a word-processor. The development of a course reader is underway but is not costed as yet.

The details in Figures 15.1-5 demonstrate convincingly that open learning is a cost effective method of delivering continuing education to nursing staff, when compared with conventional methods.

Course B

Development of the consolidation course to a distance learning mode from a totally College-based course is likely to affect course costs.
The course will be of 12 weeks duration and have 90 hours of study input from participants plus 4 in-College sessions.
Intention to offer this course 4 times per year to 20 participants in each group.

Estimated Costs:-

MATERIALS
Study packs at £25 each (3 packs per student per course)
= 240 packs   = £ 6,000

ADMINISTRATION
Secretarial time – letters – programmes – photocopying
£150 per course
for 4 courses   = £   600

TUTORIAL HOURS
4 x 3 hours study session per course =
12 hours for 4 courses = 48 hours
48 hours charged at time and a half (SN4 = £15.37)   = £   738
On costs @ 20%   = £   147

                                                                = £   885

80 hours of phone tutorial time charged at time and a half
(SN4 = £15.37)   = £ 1,229
On costs @ 20%   = £   245

                                                                £ 1,474

Total College cost of CONSOLIDATION COURSES
(distance mode)   £ 8,959

Figure 15.5 Predicted consolidation course for registered nurses

Gaining political commitment

We needed commitment at five levels. I have already discussed the process of gaining the support of educational staff in the college. Of critical concern to college staff is the economic balance of continuing income which, by definition, allows their work to continue and thereby secures ongoing employment. The myth that open learning replaces tutors is pervasive. The opposite end of this balance is the tutors' concern that they will be swamped, either by conflicting demands of conventional and distance students, or simply by large numbers of open learners. Maintaining this balance of work expectations on tutors is the central responsibility of the educational planner, particularly since there exists no simple and neat set of guidelines for maintaining an open learning programme.

The second commitment had to come from service nursing managers. They, in health services, are the users of any educational programme. The advantages to them have to be sold in terms of ease of access, no replacement of staff, and considerably reduced travel and subsistence costs.

The third commitment had to come from potential learners themselves. Students first have to be motivated into programmes which have not hitherto existed. Then they have to be persuaded that open learning programmes carry equal educational credit and last they have to be assured that they will be supported through this unfamiliar learning process.

The fourth commitment had to come from the Highland Health Board. This commitment had to be in part financial, and in part in principle. Of these two, the commitment in principle to the philosophy of open learning and the need for continuing education programmes was the more important. The contribution by the Board of £50,000 is a reflection of a commitment to the first stage of the programme.

Finally, the fifth commitment had to come from the National Board for Nursing, Midwifery and Health Visiting for Scotland. Again, the commitment had to be both in principle and financial. The commitment in principle related to maintaining the Board's agreement to mounting courses within their guidelines in an open learning format. In the event, this was easily negotiated. The financial commitment from the National Board for Scotland was reflected in the appointment to the college of a post of Senior Tutor (Open Learning).

Without any of these commitments, either in principle or in financial terms, we would not have been able to move forward.

The current position and future developments

At the time of writing, in mid-1989, the programme of implementation is being maintained to its target dates. The continuing education for Second Level Registered Nurses programme has been running since 1987, and has offered four intakes to date. The conventional Consolidation Course will be offered as planned in an open learning framework in 1989. Meanwhile, it continues to run as a conventional course until the transition date. The Diploma in Nursing, offered jointly by the Highland College and the University of London and the Distance Learning Centre commenced in September 1987. Professional Studies 1 already has some self-designed materials ready and the course will commence on target in January 1990, subject to validation by the National Board for Scotland. Finally, the tutor, counsellor and facilitator pack has been written to the first draft stage, and should be ready for use by June 1989.

Essentially, my concerns for the future relate to increasing educational provision through the college and on an open learning basis up to the millennium. Courses are required immediately for community based practitioners and a proposal for finance is being reviewed by private institutions. It is anticipated that the Diploma in Nursing already offered by the college will be extended to degree level by an add-on open learning component in the foreseeable future. Early negotiations are also in hand with a central institution to provide, again on an open learning basis, a post-registration degree in health studies with options for hospital staff, primary care staff and midwives. All of these developments will take account in their curriculum design of the currently proposed changes in the health service nationally. We will also take account of changes in educational technology and in the funding basis and accreditation systems in the education sector.

I have already drawn out the main issues for an educator who wants to change the educational system to an open learning format but in conclusion I would want to emphasise that the main issue is the importance of change being needs led. The needs of both service as a whole and the practitioner individually have to be recognised. No educational programmes offered without these prerequisites are likely to succeed. This requires a continuing dialogue with all interested parties and without this dialogue, the political and financial agreements are unlikely to be forthcoming. Student interest and uptake would most likely be low. There is a circular effect which is that, provided cooperation and negotiation are thorough, this process will lead in itself to enhanced levels of cooperation between service and education for the future, and thereby to high quality relevant educational and training provision.

References

National Board for Scotland 1985 *Guidelines for Continuing Education, Professional Studies 1 and 2.* NBS February

Scottish Home and Health Department 1981 *Continuing Education for the Nursing Profession in Scotland.* SHHD

Part 4:
Postscript

16 Postscript

Kate Robinson

This final chapter is in three parts. The first presents the paradox of the success and the failure of open learning. The second, a vision of the potential of open learning for the emancipation of nurses. The third suggests that we need to establish an ongoing debate about the role of open learning in nursing and highlights some of the important constituent parts of that debate.

The paradox

The paradox, presented briefly, is that the nursing profession urgently needs to expand its continuing education system; open learning represents a well researched and effective system of providing education on a large scale; yet the nursing profession has been slow to accept open learning as other than a minor addition to existing resources. Let me deal with each of these aspects in turn.

The profession's needs

The health care field is increasingly subject to change, and nursing has had to adapt to external changes, such as the new management structures and the use of new technology, as well as initiatives from within nursing. Nursing initiatives include the development of new therapies, for example, the so-called alternative therapies; new relationships with patients and other health care workers; an emphasis on health education; and new ways of organising care, such as primary nursing. The need for each individual to update her knowledge and skills to keep up with events has been emphasised by the United Kingdom Central Council (UKCC), and the Code of Professional Conduct (UKCC 1984) demands that they do it as a matter of urgency.

Despite this enormous need there is extensive evidence that the opportunities for professional development are limited (Rogers and Lawrence 1987; Lathlean 1988).

The claims of open learning

The arguments for open learning have been rehearsed in previous chapters, which drew on some of the research evidence on open learning. A brief perusal of the pages of the journal *Open Learning* shows that there is a large body of research evidence about many facets of open learning. Admittedly much of this research relates to academic rather than vocational learning, and little of it applies directly to health care or nursing. However, it shows that open learning is a useful, complex and effective educational methodology.

If we look to countries abroad, we can find numerous accounts of open learning in nursing being used successfully. For example, open learning for nurse education was a major theme in presentations from the USA and Canada for the conference *Pathways for Progress* hosted by the University of Wales School of Nursing Studies 1988 and developments have been reported elsewhere (*see*, for example, Kerr 1988). Similarly, Australia and New Zealand, have used open learning for nursing for some years; indeed much of the inspiration for the Distance Learning Centre came from a sabbatical spent by Sheila Jackson, formerly education officer of the English National Board, at a specialist centre producing open learning courses in Australia. Some of the developments in open learning in Australia and New Zealand with reference to nursing education have been written up by Chick and Paull (1988). Nearer to home, open learning plays an important part in nurse education in Sweden, where there are a number of courses in topics like nursing research and nurse education.

The progress of open learning

To say that open learning has progressed faster or slower than expected is a value judgement dependent on the expectations of the individual, and enthusiasts probably want faster progress than is reasonable. A case could be made that enormous progress has been made since, say, 1984 when *A Systematic Approach to Nursing Care* was published by the Open University. By any one of a number of reasonable criteria there have been exciting initiatives, for example, the English National Board has approved both open learning and mixed mode courses; the Department of Health has funded a major research project on open learning in nursing; the English National Board is developing its own materials and has financed further exploratory work in open learning; the Health Pickup programme is set to produce an extensive series of packs for nurses and others; the National Board for Scotland is working with the Highland College of

Nursing and Midwifery to promote open learning and the Welsh Board has encouraged the use of Teaching and Assessing Nurses (Distance Learning Centre 1985) within its approved courses. This list could be extended, and indeed many of the chapters in Part Three looked at local initiatives.

However, the research evidence (Lawrence *et al* 1988), and anecdotal evidence from the producers of open learning materials and others (*see*, for example, Price 1989), indicate that open learning is not established within nurse education in general, and has only a foothold within continuing education.

This is in contrast with experience in other similar occupations where open learning has been a more important part of education. For example, open learning has been central to continuing education for the teaching profession; the Open University from its foundation specifically targeted teachers and has a School of Education producing courses at undergraduate and masters degree level, as well as shorter updating packs. Within social work, open learning has been used for updating but it also has a place in basic training; the Open University has worked with the Central Council for Education and Training in Social Work (CCETSW) to evolve courses which can be credited both by CCETSW and by the Open University. The production of P553 *A Systematic Approach to Nursing Care* by the Open University could have been seen as the beginning of a similar partnership between the nursing profession and the University but the initiative was not followed up on either side until the late 1980s. Similarly, the establishment of two Open Tech projects for nursing (the Distance Learning Centre and Continuing Nurse Education Programme) could have been grasped as the major opportunity to move forward with open learning but, although both projects have survived, neither could be said to prosper.

Explaining the paradox

How can this paradox be explained? There are a number of ways of explaining why open learning has yet to make the impact on nursing which might reasonably have been predicted. Price (1989), for example, details some of the problems encountered by tutors in using learning materials, such as the difficulties of integrating them with their own teaching and the lack of time for reviewing what was available. A more general explanation lies in the profession's interest in other matters throughout the 1980s; the establishment of the statutory bodies and the development of Project 2000 took a great deal of the energy and enthusiasm which might have reasonably underpinned the movement into open learning. Open learning has been seen mainly in the context of continuing education and this is the area of nurse education which has, in some parts of the UK, lacked direction and purpose. It may be that the advantages of open learning cannot be specified in an area where so little is known about the function, purpose and shape of the educational process. The future of open learning seems therefore to be inextricably linked with the development of the philosophy and organisation of continuing education: the directors of both the Distance Learning Centre and the Continuing Nurse Education Programme realised early on that their eventual success depended in large measure on a definitive statement on mandatory refreshment coming from the statutory bodies. The adoption of open learning – an innovation within nursing, even if well established elsewhere – depends on it being seen as a solution to the problem of providing appropriate continuing education for the large and scattered nursing workforce. But until the introduction of *mandatory* refreshment, then there is no felt need; continuing education is a luxury item with very little resource allocation. This argument explains both the general lack of growth of open learning and also the success of particular open learning items – *A Systematic Approach to Nursing Care* (Open University 1984) was successful because adoption of the nursing process was essential for any training establishment; the success of *Teaching and Assessing Nurses* (DLC 1985) was linked to the introduction of the National Board Teaching and Assessing courses. Similarly, open learning will become important within return to practice courses and second to first level conversion courses because of explicit needs generated by the statutory bodies.

My conclusion, therefore, is that open learning clearly has a place in continuing education but that place reflects the insignificance currently afforded to continuing education. However, assuming that continuing education grows rapidly in the future, open learning will contribute greatly to nurse education, but that contribution could take various forms. I want to propose that it could make a particular contribution to creating the independent nurse practitioner of the future if the full potential of open learning is realised.

A vision of emancipation

We can propose two distinct functions for continuing education. *First,* to maintain the skills of a large and scattered workforce in a setting in which technology and organisation is ever changing, and *second,* the development of the individual nurse into the 'knowledgeable doer' able to play a full role in the care of individuals with complex problems and in development of the health services to meet the challenge of health needs. The latter is obviously derived from the prescription in Project 2000 (UKCC 1987), while the former probably relates more closely to the aims of management. Open learning can play a major role in both aspects, but it will be a different sort of open learning emphasising different aspects of the educational process. In the words of Snell *et al* (1987), it can be used for *dissemination* or *development.*

In terms of the justification for open learning, the concepts of dissemination or development tend to be translated into arguments about quantity or quality, and those in favour of open learning in nursing have been mainly about quantity – '*see how many more people can be sent on a course for the same money*' – rather than quality. The *quality* of open learning relates to the learning experience, and within a vocational area this experience should enhance the sort of competencies required for practice. That is to say, the learners should utilise the same sort of skills and abilities within the educational programme that they will be asked to exercise in their work.

If we consider the possibilities within education, we could use open learning to promote a nurse who could quickly master new skills in order to extend her role at short notice, either because of staff shortages, a move to a new area or the introduction of new technology. Or we could produce a programme which offered a high degree of complexity and uncertainty and developed the ability of the nurse to solve complex problems in real situations. Clearly that sort of independent problem-solving matches the style and competence envisaged for the new practitioners of Project 2000.

I want to expand this theme by using concepts drawn from an analysis of open learning in a different situation (Farnes 1988); the two concepts are *emancipation* and *domestication*. Farnes reports on a scheme for offering open learning activities to mothers with young children living in deprived environments who could not or would not normally become involved in education. They are domesticated by their social situation; being isolated from each other and from the community because they have young children, and they are handicapped in overcoming their situation by a lack of resources. It seems to me that the situation of many nurses is similarly 'domesticated', by which I am not referring to their home situation – although this may be a contributing factor to their problems – but to the fact that they are often isolated in the work situation by geography, by lack of staff, by shiftwork, and that they have few resources with which to remedy their situation.

Farnes, reporting on the success of the open learning programme provided for the women, found that:

- participation was encouraged by the provision of appropriate resources, ie child care, learning materials, group leaders, other students and convenient facilities

- learning appeared to contribute to the resources of students in that they gain knowledge and skills, extend their social networks, and enjoy improved self-esteem and confidence
- some students use these increased resources to engage in new activities and make changes which extend beyond their domestic lives into the community
- many of the students report the resources gained from learning, the subsequent changes and new activities in terms which suggest that they experience an increase in emancipation.

I do not think it is too far fetched to view the nursing occupation as one which has been domesticated and which requires emancipation. Emancipation within nursing could be promoted if the conditions described by Farnes could be reproduced, that is, if courses were provided and properly resourced. The learning that would go on in such situations would allow the participants, like those in Farnes' study, to become more active in other parts of their working and private lives and in places other than their immediate environment.

The receptive learner

Despite the obvious advantages of emancipation through open learning, it is not always welcomed by the potential audience – not all slaves wanted to be free! Within nursing, this reluctance may be partly because they believe it will necessitate using more of their leisure time as study time at work is cut down. This is, of course, a side effect of open learning rather than an intrinsic component. Nevertheless, it is a real fear: students of mine have considered transferring from the Open University to a local face-to-face course simply to get the study leave which is otherwise denied to them. However, there are other reasons for the learners' rejection of open learning which are more profound and more worrying. It is difficult to reconcile the often heard statement that '*open learning is fine for some people, but I couldn't manage it – I am not good at working on my own*' with the idea of an independent practitioner. After all, if she can't manage a carefully constructed, well supported open learning course, then how will she manage the independent literature searching and collating of information which is involved in knowledgeable practice? Such a learner has not learnt how to learn despite (or because of?) many years in conventional education. Open learning is not just for the well motivated – it is a way of *teaching* self-motivation and self-awareness. Learners who practise organising and structuring their own learning may learn the skills necessary for them to act on their own working environment.

Control

One danger of a movement into open learning is that the dependence on centrally produced materials could lead to a homogeneous culture becoming more widespread within nursing. Earlier chapters have highlighted the real danger of materials providing one message and John Paley's account illustrates well how racism and sexism can be conveyed by materials produced by the most well meaning of course teams. British culture, and therefore nursing, is essentially segmented over health as over other issues and this needs to be reflected in each nurse's learning experience. The other side of the coin is that open learning materials, particularly audio and video-tape, offer the nurse a much broader view of culture than could be provided within one school or college. Quality, therefore, needs to be related to a multidimensional approach.

The debate

Throughout this book a number of issues and questions have been raised with no conclusive answer given. This is appropriate given the innovatory nature of open learning with nursing; to prescribe answers to questions which have not yet been widely discussed would be premature. The main purpose of this book, however, has been to provide information for the debate on the nature and purpose of open learning which should take place in nursing in the next decade. That debate will cover all the aspects dealt with in previous chapters and probably many more.

There is a danger, however, that the debate will not be concerned with the issues of quality in open learning but with the *control* of open learning. Both the statutory bodies and the National Health Service Training Authority (NHSTA) are making major investments in open learning for nurse training, although the NHSTA initiatives are directed at nurses *and* other care groups. Inevitably their approaches will differ and these differences will need to be explored in the evaluation of the programmes in a constructive way. Open learning is a broad church and there is room for many models to be used to accommodate different needs. A polarisation of opinion along political lines would not, however, be useful for the learners. The following issues, however, are central to the experience of the learner.

The teachers

The role of the teacher in open learning is not, of course, a lesser role, which was a fear expressed in the early stages of the Open Tech programme, but it is different and may require considerable change in the way we train and use teachers. It may be that resistance to change comes because open learning is tacked onto existing responsibilities as an extra task; in this situation the teacher does not have the time to either choose the most appropriate learning materials and integrate them into a curriculum, or offer appropriate support to learners. Price (1989) proposes the solution:

> Schools of nursing and postbasic tutors may have to demand breathing space to review and select, so that packages can be brought down off the shelf and put into action.

The resources

Clearly open learning requires that resources are distributed in a different fashion. Costs are skewed towards production, either in direct costs or through purchase of materials, and the maintenance costs of the system, that is the administrative and support systems, should be less costly than in conventional teaching. This would require a substantial change in the funding system for pre-registration training; for post-registration training the funding base is generally so low that almost any initiative is going to require an increase in resources. In this context Chris Wakeling's detailed information on the funding of her scheme (Chapter 15) is extremely welcome. However, open learning does *not* provide a low cost answer to education – although it is cost-effective, mainly because of savings in peripheral costs such as travel time. Some savings may be made by transferring the costs to the learner. The lure of cheap education was behind some of the Open Tech initiatives but the programme showed conclusively that, as in other areas of life, you get what you pay for:

> Open learning provision is like other MSC projects: they want it quickly, cheaply and of good quality. Nobody can score more than two out of those three.
>
> Open University 1988

Credit accumulation and transfer

Credit accumulation and transfer schemes offer viable frameworks for open learning programmes which are usually organised into small units of learning. Such schemes allow learning to be split into small elements which are assessed and the credit gained can be carried forward either within the same course or into different courses. Conventionally organised linear curricula such as the Diploma in Nursing (University of London) inhibit an open learning scheme from providing the flexibility to the learner which is one of the great strengths of open learning. As credit accumulation and transfer schemes become more widespread, the use of open learning modules within them for all or part of the learning process may also be extended. However, it is important that the use of open learning in this context is anticipated and regulations do not inadvertently preclude it by, for example, specifying study in a classroom, or consecutive days of study. Similarly, producers of open learning modules must make sure that learners have the information necessary for them to apply for credit within, for example, the development of professional practice framework of the Welsh National Board. This scheme encourages credit accumulation and transfer, but learners need to apply individually:

> Students seeking accreditation of other courses, eg Open University credits, for inclusion in the award, should apply directly to the Welsh National Board giving all the relevant information and documentary proof of successful completion.
> To apply for credit exemptions, full details of courses completed, with documentary evidence of successful completion, must be submitted on an individual basis.
>
> WNB 1989

Evaluation

No debate on an educational initiative would be complete without a focus on evaluation and the dangers of over-enthusiastic innovation in open learning have been noticed:

> Unfortunately, the field is so new that standards of quality have not yet been laid down. Consequently, it is not easy for users to tell the difference between the experienced and competent providers of Open Learning and those whose enthusiasm outruns their competence and whose ignorant or exploitative approach to Open Learning might bring the whole idea into disrepute. It would not be the first innovation where bad practices have driven out the good.
>
> MSC 1988

Within open learning there are different aspects to evaluation and different mechanisms; for example, the learning materials need to be evaluated in production as well as in use (*see* Chapter 3). However, the processes of evaluating open learning have been well documented and there are many precedents for nursing to draw on (*see,* for example, Thorpe 1988). Thorpe warns of the danger that evaluation becomes reduced to quality control according to some specified model or design. Such a model might say, for example, that learning materials *must include* objectives. This danger is inherent in prescriptions for quality such as the code of practice for open learning (MSC 1988), which should therefore be used with care. Open learning in nursing needs room to develop a number of different modes and models within an evaluation framework which emphasises the importance both of the learner's experience and the consequences for patient care.

A forum for the debate?

The debate about open learning in nursing is already underway at a number of levels; for example, the nursing press has explored the issues. However, it may be that to take the debate forward in a fully constructive manner a more explicit structure is required. A number of the projects within the Open Tech programme formed the Open Learning Forum for the Caring Professions which had the following objectives:

- liaison with accreditation agencies
- providing information and consultancy on open learning to the health care market
- establishing joint projects, including those to extend existing materials and produce new materials, distribution projects for open learning projects and services, and spreading the experience gained in setting up open learning programmes.

Although the forum held a number of useful meetings in 1985/6 it could not continue because of lack of funding. A resurrected forum, which was open to all the interested parties both within and without nursing, including for example the relevant validating bodies, could perform a useful coordinating and liaison role as well as stimulating the kind of debate which has been outlines here.

References

Chick N and Paull D 1988 Collaboration between nurse educators in Australia and New Zealand extends educational opportunities for nurses. *International Journal of Nursing Studies* 25 4 pp279-86

DLC 1985 *Teaching and Assessing Nurses*. Distance Learning Centre

Farnes N 1988 Open University Community Education: emancipation or domestication *Open Learning* 3 1 pp35-40

Kerr J R 1988 Nursing education at a distance: using technology to advantage in undergraduate and graduate degree programs in Alberta, Canada. *International Journal of Nursing Studies* 25, 4 pp301-6

Lathlean J 1988 Policy issues in continuing education for clinical nurses in White R (ed.) *Political Issues in Nursing* John Wiley

Lawrence J, Maggs C, Rogers J 1988 Interim Report on an Evaluation of the Use of Distance Learning Materials for Continuing Professional Education for Qualified Nurses, Midwives and Health Visitors. Istitute of Education. University of London

MSC 1988 *Ensuring Quality in Open Learning: a handbook for action.* Manpower Services Commission

Open University 1988 Module 2 *Open Learning.*The Open University Press

Price B 1989 Left on the shelf? *Nursing Times* 85 *19* p71

Rogers J and Lawrence J 1987 *Continuing Professional Education for Qualified Nurses, Midwives and Health Visitors: a report of a survey and case study.* Institute of Education, Ashdale Press and Austen Cornish

Snell R S, Hodgson V E, Mann S J 1987 Beyond distance teaching towards open learning. In Hodgson V E, Mann S J and Snell R S (eds) *Beyond Distance teaching – Towards Open Learning* The Society for Research into Higher Education and Open University Press

Thorpe M 1988 *Evaluating Open and Distance Learning.* Longman

UKCC 1984 *Code of Professional Conduct for the Nurse, Midwife and Health Visitor.* United Kingdom Central Council

UKCC 1987 *Project 2000: The Final Proposals.* United Kingdom Central Council for Nursing Midwifery and Health Visiting

WNB 1989 *The Development of Professional Practice.* Welsh National Board

Further reading

Open Learning is the major journal concerned with open learning within the UK; it is published three times a year by Longman

Bates A W (ed.) 1984 *The Role of Technology in Distance Education.* Croom Helm

Dixon K 1987 *Implementing Open Learning in Local Authority Institutions* Further Education Unit/Open Learning Branch of the Manpower Services Commission, 2nd edition

Hodgson V E , Mann S J and Snell R (eds.) 1987 *Beyond Distance Teaching - Towards Open Learning.* Society for Research into Higher Education and Open University Press

Keegan D 1986 *The Foundations of Distance Education.* Croom Helm

Lawrence J, Maggs C, Rogers J 1988 *Interim Report on an Evaluation of the Use of Distance Learning Materials for Continuing Professional Education for Qualified Nurses, Midwives and Health Visitors.* Institute of Education, University of London

Lewis R 1984 *Open Learning in Action.* Council for Educational Technology

Marson S *Teachers' Guide to Open/Distance Learning.* ENB Learning Resources Unit, Sheffield

MSC 1988 *Ensuring Quality in Open Learning: a Handbook for Action.* Manpower Services Commission

OU 1988 Open Learning Module 2 *Professional Studies in Post-Compulsory Education* DO5 Part B/E86. The Open University Press

Paine N (ed.) 1988 *Open Learning in Transition.* National Extension College

Perry W 1976 *Open University.* The Open University Press

Rogers J, Maggs C, Lawrence J 1989 *Distance Learning Materials for Continuing Professional Education for Qualified Nurses, Midwives and Health Visitors.* A report of a survey and evaluation. Institute of Education, University of London

Thorpe M and Grugeon D (eds.) 1987 *Open Learning for Adults.* Longman

Thorpe M 1988 *Evaluating Open and Distance Learning.* Longman

Woolfe R, Murgatroyd S, Rhys S 1987 *Guidance and Counselling in Adult and Continuing Education.* The Open University Press